HAIRDRESSING SCIENCE
THIRD EDITION

HAIRDRESSING SCIENCE

(third edition)

Florence Openshaw, BSc., MIT

An imprint of **Pearson Education**

Harlow, England · London · New York · Reading, Massachusetts · San Francisco
Toronto · Don Mills, Ontario · Sydney · Tokyo · Singapore · Hong Kong · Seoul
Taipei · Cape Town · Madrid · Mexico City · Amsterdam · Munich · Paris · Milan

Pearson Education Limited
Edinburgh Gate
Harlow
Essex CM20 2JE
England

and Associated Companies throughout the world

Visit us on the World Wide Web at:
http://www.pearsoned.co.uk

First published 1978
Second edition 1986
Third edition 1995

British Library Cataloguing in Publication Data
A catalogue entry for this title is available from the British Library.

ISBN 0-582-24197-9

10   9   8
07   06   05   04   03

Set by 4 in 10/12 Plantin
Printed in Malaysia, GPS

CONTENTS

PREFACE TO THE THIRD EDITION

For this third edition of *Hairdressing Science* the text has been completely reviewed and updated to follow the scheme set out by the Hairdressing Training Board for the National Vocational Qualifications Level 2 in Hairdressing. A change of emphasis reflects the growing concern for the safe use of chemicals and the assessment of health hazards. Throughout the book students are alerted to the effects of the misapplication of chemical products and the misuse of appliances.

Features of this edition include a new section on Afro hairdressing, considerable expansion of chapters on hair condition and the use of conditioning treatments, a glossary for quick reference and the addition of groups of questions for student self testing. In one important respect the book has not changed. Science is still integrated closely with hairdressing and in this way the relevance of science to hairdressing is maintained.

Once again I wish to express my thanks to my former colleague, John Eaton, of Nelson and Colne College for valuable technical discussions, information and advice.

ACKNOWLEDGEMENTS

We are indebted to the following people for permission to reproduce copyright material:

Dr Tony Brain/Science Photo Library: Fig. 8.11
Chubb Fire Ltd: Fig. 4.2
J. A. Crabtree Ltd: Figs 5.9, 5.13
Dimplex Heating Ltd: Figs. 2.8a, 2.9a
Eastern Electricity: Fig. 2.10a
GE Lighting: Figs 2.18, 2.19a, 2.19b, 2.21
Houseman Hegro, Permutit Domestic Division: Figs 12.7a, b, 12.10b
Institute of Dermatology: Figs 1.9, 8.12
Dr P. Marazzi/Science Photo Library: Fig. 8.10
Remington: Fig. 13.8
Suter: Fig. 11.3
C. James Webb: Fig. 3.3
Wella International: Figs 6.3b, 9.1
Carole Wright/Format: Fig. 16.2

While every effort has been made to trace the owners of copyright material, in a few cases this has proved impossible and we take the opportunity to offer our apologies to any copyright holders whose rights we may have unwittingly infringed.

PART 1
HEALTH AND SAFETY

1

THE HAIRDRESSER: APPEARANCE AND PERSONAL HYGIENE

It is important for the running of a successful hairdressing business that clients obtain a favourable impression of both the salon and its staff. In addition to the cultivation of a professional attitude towards the client, hairdressers must also consider their own personal appearance and deportment. Particular attention should be paid to personal hygiene.

Hairdressers often work in conditions which are far from ideal. They tend to stand for long hours, and are thus subject to foot troubles which may lead to bad posture and fatigue. Unless the ventilation is good, the salon may become too hot and humid, making the hairdresser perspire freely and become uncomfortable and irritable. Many of the substances used are damaging to the skin, the hands particularly being at risk, and special care must be taken to keep them in good condition. Clients notice the state of the hairdresser's skin, nails, hair and clothing. It is essential not only to have a clean and tidy salon, but also that hairdressers themselves present a well-groomed appearance and avoid giving offence to clients by perspiration or breath odours.

POSTURE

Bad posture can lead to both fatigue and lasting ill-health if strain is placed on muscles and ligaments, and if respiration and circulation are restricted by rounded shoulders causing compression of the chest. In addition, bad posture gives the client an impression of an unenthusiastic and careless worker. Clothes, too, do not look their best, and may hang unevenly, for they are made to fit a well-balanced figure.

Posture is dependent on the skeleton, the ligaments which bind the bones together and the muscles which enable movement to take place.

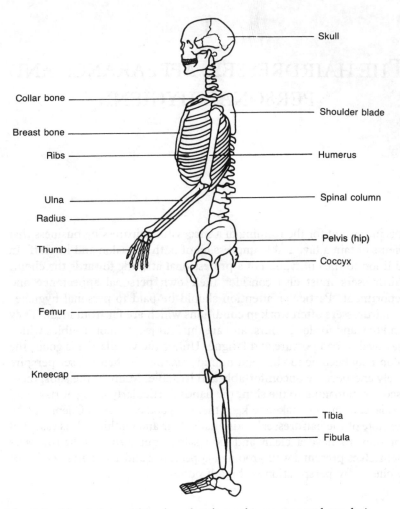

Fig. 1.1 The skeleton (side view showing only one arm and one leg)

The skeleton

The skeleton is shown in Fig. 1.1. It has several important functions:

- to support the body, giving it a rigid structure and enabling it to keep its shape
- to support internal organs, e.g. the pelvis supports the abdominal organs
- to protect delicate organs, e.g. the rib-cage protects the heart and lungs; the skull protects the brain

- to form a point of attachment for muscles enabling movement to take place.

Ligaments

The ligaments, which strap the adjacent bones together, are pliable and allow movement at the joints. In bad posture it is often the ligaments which suffer strain by being overstretched. The position of the ligaments can be seen in the **hinge joint** in Fig. 1.2. This type of joint, found at the elbow and knee, allows movement in one direction only. Other types of movable joint are the **ball and socket joint** found at the hips and shoulders, and the **plane or gliding joint** in which two flat surfaces move over each other, as in the wrist and the spine.

Muscles

Muscles are attached to bones by tendons which are non-elastic. When the muscles contract, the bones are pulled into a different position, as for example the movement of the forearm (see Fig. 1.3). Contraction of the biceps raises the forearm. Contraction of the triceps straightens the arm.

Muscles are always in a state of slight contraction, ready to respond when movement is required. This condition is known as **muscle tone**. The contraction of muscle needs energy which is obtained chemically by the oxidation of the glucose brought to the muscle in the bloodstream,

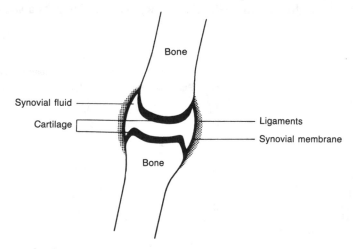

Fig. 1.2 Section through a hinge joint

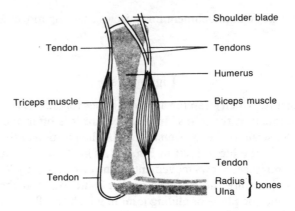

Shoulder blade

Tendon

Tendons

Humerus

Triceps muscle

Biceps muscle

Tendon

Tendon

Tendon

Radius } bones
Ulna }

Fig. 1.3 Muscle action

and stored there until required. During exercise, increase in heart rate and in breathing rate bring extra supplies of glucose and oxygen to the muscles. **Muscle fatigue** results if waste products accumulate in the muscle, and resting is required to allow recovery.

Posture while standing

Posture is correct if a straight line can be drawn from the mastoid bone just behind the ear, through the tip of the shoulder, through the middle line of the hips, to the front of the knee and the front of the ankle (see Fig. 1.4). **Posture fatigue** is caused when one part of the body is out of line with the part immediately below, because this puts a strain on

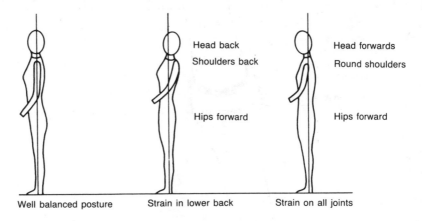

Head back
Shoulders back

Head forwards
Round shoulders

Hips forward

Hips forward

Well balanced posture   Strain in lower back   Strain on all joints

Fig. 1.4 Posture (forwards-and-backwards plane)

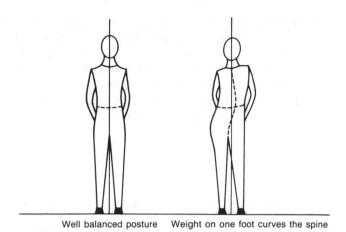

Well balanced posture   Weight on one foot curves the spine

Fig. 1.5 Posture (sideways plane)

the ligaments. Balance must be maintained in a forward-and-backward plane and also in a sideways plane (see Fig. 1.5).

If, as in hairdressing, it is necessary to stand for long periods, a change of position is often restful. To habitually stand with the weight on one foot strains the ligaments in the spine (see Fig. 1.5), but the leg muscles can be rested alternately for short periods. Normally the feet should be a little distance apart so that the legs are vertical or straight down from the hips. The toes should point straight forwards both in standing and walking, so that the body weight falls on the flat outer edges of the feet and not on the arches.

The shoulders should be level and point straight out to the sides. If the left shoulder is higher than the right, the lower spine bends to the left and the ligaments on the left side of the spine become stretched. If the shoulders are brought forwards, the chest is compressed and the upper part of the back is rounded, so stretching the back muscles and ligaments. If the shoulders are pushed too far back, the natural curve of the back is flattened and this causes tension.

The head should be held straight up. If the chin drops, the line of vision is changed. If the chin is pushed outwards, the head tilts back causing strain in the neck and shoulder muscles. Holding the head on one side causes tension in the neck and shoulder muscles, as well as affecting vision as the eyes are on different levels.

Posture while sitting

In order that sitting should be restful, the back should be supported all the way down by sitting well back in the chair. There should be right angles at both hips and knees so that no tension occurs in the joints. The weight of the body should be supported by the pelvis and not by the bottom of the spine. Some of the weight of the thighs should be supported by the feet or there will be pressure on the blood vessels and nerves at the back of the thighs. Sitting with one leg over the other can result in similar pressure, and this may impair circulation causing the limb to 'go to sleep' or have 'pins and needles'.

FATIGUE

Different forms of fatigue may be experienced by the hairdresser:

- **Muscular fatigue** caused by prolonged working, which results in aching muscles and slowness of movement.
- **Posture fatigue** due to strain on the muscles and ligaments by bad posture.
- **Mental fatigue** due to prolonged mental activity results in frequent mistakes and forgetfulness.
- **Heat fatigue** due to working in a hot, stuffy atmosphere may lead to headaches, dizziness or fainting.

Hairdressers spend a long time on their feet, and so periods of rest with the feet raised are beneficial, along with adequate sleep and rest at night. Some form of outdoor exercise is necessary and will improve respiration and circulation, as well as relaxing nervous tension.

CARE OF THE FEET

Special care of the feet is required to avoid discomfort which may affect posture and the ability to stand and walk correctly. A chiropodist should be consulted if any painful conditions arise.

The following foot conditions may need attention.

- **Corns** are a thickening of the epidermis (the outer layer of the skin) due to pressure by ill-fitting shoes.
- **Ingrowing toe nails** result from pressure on the nails. The condition may be eased by cutting the nails straight across or slightly concave.
- **Bunions** (Hallux Vulgus) are caused by incorrectly fitting shoes. The joint of the big toe becomes inflamed, causing pain and resulting in an unsightly shaped foot.
- **Flat feet** (Pes planus) and fallen arches (see Fig. 1.6) may be due to

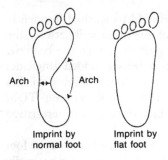

Fig. 1.6   Flat feet

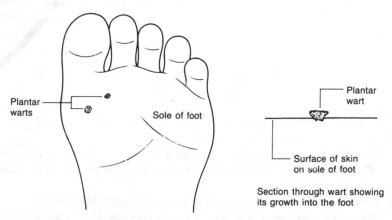

Fig. 1.7   Plantar warts

continual standing or may be inherited. The arches of the foot are maintained by strong ligaments which are prevented from stretching by the muscles in the legs. Strain and tiredness of these muscles can result in fallen arches. The condition may be treated by exercise or by artificial support to the arches.

- **Plantar warts** (verrucae) (see Fig. 1.7) are a form of ingrowing wart on the sole of the foot and may be painful due to pressure when walking. They are caused by a viral infection which may be picked up when walking barefoot in public places such as at swimming pools. Verrucae may be treated by a chiropodist.
- **Calluses** are patches of hard skin caused by shoe friction on the sole of the foot. They may be due to bad posture when the body's weight is not evenly distributed.
- **Athlete's foot** is a fungus infection resulting in soggy white patches between the toes. Medical attention is required.

The above conditions can largely be avoided by attention to foot hygiene and the use of correct footwear. The feet should be washed frequently especially if they perspire freely. They should be dried well between the toes, as warmth and moisture encourage the growth of fungi and bacteria. Dusting the feet with foot powder (talcum powder with added fungicide) will help absorb sweat and prevent the growth of fungi. Wiping the feet with cologne or surgical spirit is also helpful to control sweating. Tight shoes and tight socks, stockings or tights, which cause lack of ventilation to the feet, should be avoided.

Shoes should grip at the heel and over the instep. The arch of the foot should be supported and there should be room for the toes to move easily inside the shoe. Very high heels tend to throw the body forward and this leads to bad posture. Claw toes may result if the foot slips forward in the shoe due to high heels. A low or medium heel is usually more comfortable.

SELF TESTING

1. Why is personal appearance so important for a hairdresser?
2. What is the cause of posture fatigue?
3. Describe the correct posture for a hairdresser when standing at work.
4. What is the effect of habitually standing with the weight on one foot only?
5. Describe the correct posture for a receptionist when seated.
6. What different forms of fatigue may be experienced by a hairdresser?
7. What may cause (a) corns (b) calluses (c) plantar warts (d) athlete's foot?
8. What steps can be taken to treat excessive foot perspiration?
9. What is the effect of wearing (a) tight shoes (b) very high heels?

PERSONAL HYGIENE

Careful attention to personal hygiene is essential both for the health of the individual hairdresser and to avoid offence to the client.

Care of the skin

Unpleasant body odour results from the breakdown of perspiration by bacteria and is associated with those areas of the body, such as the axillae (underarms), the genital area, and the feet, where there is least ventilation of the skin. Perspiration is produced by sweat glands lying in the skin, each gland having a duct through which sweat passes to the skin surface.

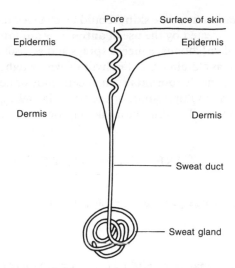

Pore   Surface of skin

Epidermis   Epidermis

Dermis   Dermis

Sweat duct

Sweat gland

Fig. 1.8 Eccrine sweat gland

There are two types of sweat glands in the skin: eccrine and apocrine glands.

Eccrine or sudoriferous glands

The eccrine or sudoriferous glands (see Fig. 1.8) are found practically all over the surface of the body. They secrete perspiration consisting of salt (2 per cent) and water (98 per cent) with traces of waste products such as urea and lactic acid.

In temperate climates, about 1 litre of eccrine sweat is secreted per day without the skin becoming wet. This is known as **insensible perspiration**. The secretion of perspiration is increased by heat and nervous tension.

Apocrine or odoriferous glands

The apocrine or odoriferous glands are found mostly in the armpits. They are generally larger than the eccrine glands and secrete sweat with a greater content of fat. This type of perspiration is more readily broken down by bacteria, resulting in unpleasant body odour.

Dealing with perspiration

A daily bath or shower is necessary to remove both types of sweat along with dead skin cells, dirt, bacteria, and excess sebum (an oil produced by the sebaceous glands in the skin). Underclothing, which readily absorbs perspiration from the skin, should be changed daily. Underarm sweating may be treated by the use of **antiperspirant lotions**, which are packaged as 'roll on' lotions, squeeze sprays and aerosols. They contain **astringents** such as aluminium chlorohydrate which tighten the skin and reduce sweating, and **deodorants** such as cetrimide or hexachlorophane which prevent the multiplication of the bacteria causing odour by the breakdown of sweat. Dusting with talcum powder is also helpful.

CARE OF THE HANDS

The skin of the hands presents special problems.

Contact dermatitis

Contact dermatitis may be caused by certain substances commonly used in hairdressing such as para dyes (in permanent tints), ammonium thioglycollate (in perm lotion), lanolin (used in conditioners) and sodium lauryl sulphate in some soapless shampoos. Dermatitis (see Fig. 1.9) is an inflammation of the skin caused by contact with an irritant substance. A **primary irritant** causes inflammation on its first contact with the skin. A **secondary irritant** or **sensitizer** causes inflammation only in certain people who have already had previous contact with the substance without ill effect. They are then said to be **allergic** to the substance and further contact must be avoided. The symptoms due to an allergic reaction appear a few hours after contact with the substance and may last for several days. They may be mild with slight reddening of the skin, or may result in serious swelling of the tissues or blistering and cracking of the skin. To avoid contact dermatitis, hairdressers should always wear protective gloves when applying para dyes or perm lotion. (Clients must also be protected against dermatitis by having a skin test to ensure that para dyes can safely be applied.)

Shampoo dermatitis

A hairdresser's hands may also be affected by the continual use of water and detergents during shampooing. Soapless shampoos, the types of shampoo now most commonly used, tend to remove sebum (the natural oil of the skin) from the skin's surface. This oily layer of sebum normally keeps the skin supple by helping to retain sufficient moisture in the outer layer of the skin to enable it to stretch and wrinkle without cracking. Lack of sebum enables additional water to enter the skin causing it to

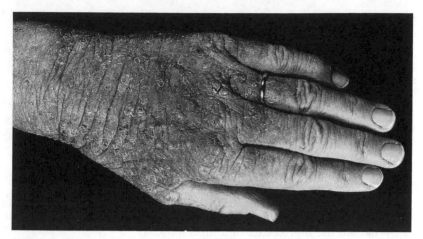

Fig. 1.9 Contact dermatitis

swell and later become rough and chapped, a condition known as shampoo dermatitis. Bacteria may enter the cracks causing infection. Hands should be rinsed thoroughly after shampooing, especially the area between the fingers and under rings, though the latter are best removed before starting to shampoo. Hand cream regularly applied, particularly at night, will help to replace the oily film on the skin and keep the hands in good condition.

Nails

Nails should be kept clean and well manicured. Dirty or badly bitten nails give a bad impression to the clients and dirt under the nails is a breeding ground for bacteria. Nails should be of a practical length and kept very smooth so as not to scratch the client's scalp or catch on the client's hair. Strong detergents remove oil from nails, leaving them brittle. Nail enamel offers some protection against this loss of oil.

ORAL HYGIENE

Unpleasant breath (halitosis), which can cause offence to clients, may result from digestive problems or from particles of food lodged in decaying teeth or in pockets between the teeth and gums. These particles are often difficult to remove by brushing and dental advice is required.

Offence to clients can also be caused by the lingering smell of tobacco smoke or by eating strong-smelling foods such as oranges, garlic, raw onions and highly spiced foods.

Mouth hygiene (oral hygiene) involves frequent cleansing of the teeth, regular visits to the dentist and sometimes, if necessary, the use of antiseptic mouthwashes.

SELF TESTING

1. How is unpleasant body odour produced?
2. Where are the apocrine glands situated?
3. What steps can be taken to prevent body odour?
4. What is an astringent?
5. What are the ingredients of antiperspirants?
6. Why are protective gloves required when applying perm lotion?
7. What is meant by 'shampoo dermatitis'?
8. How can shampoo dermatitis be avoided?
9. Why should a hairdresser's nails be short and smooth?
10. What is meant by 'halitosis'?
11. What are the causes of halitosis?
12. Name three foods which may cause offensive breath odours.

CLOTHING FOR SALON WEAR

- Clean clothing should be worn each day.
- Clothing should be loose fitting to allow easy circulation of air around the body.
- Clothing should never impede the movement of the wearer, nor interfere with the circulation by being too tight at any point.
- Very loose sleeves should be avoided because they may transfer infection from salon surfaces to the client's hair.
- Avoid belts with looped ends which may lead to accidents by catching on furniture.
- Avoid dangling jewellery or rings which may scratch clients or catch on their hair.
- Overalls or outerwear for the salon should be water-repellent in case of accidental splashing during shampooing. They should also be resistant to dirt, creases and the chemicals used in the salon.
- Nylon, while easy to launder, is uncomfortable for salon wear as it retains body heat and increases sweating. Cotton/polyester overalls

are cool and comfortable though slightly more difficult to launder than nylon.

First impressions

A well-groomed hairdresser, with neat and tidy hair, immaculately dressed and maintaining good posture, creates an immediate impression of efficiency and this at the same time improves the hairdresser's own self-confidence. Such a hairdresser is a good advertisement for the salon.

2

THE SALON: HEALTHY WORKING CONDITIONS

In order to ensure the health and comfort of both staff and clients, hairdressing salons must always be warm, well ventilated, adequately lit and kept clean. Regulations governing these conditions are laid down in the Workplace (Health, Safety and Welfare) Regulations 1992. The cleanliness of the salon will be considered in Chapter 3.

WARMTH AND VENTILATION

Efficient control of heating and ventilation systems is required to maintain comfortable air conditions in the salon. Changes in temperature, in the amount of moisture in the air (the humidity), and in the amount of movement of the air may upset the normal mechanism by which the human body keeps at a constant temperature of 36.9°C. Discomfort may result from overheating or from excessive cooling. If the air in a busy salon is not changed frequently, humidity and fumes, for example from perm lotions and hair sprays, may lead to stuffiness and the occupants may feel tired or faint.

REGULATION OF BODY TEMPERATURE

The body attempts to keep its own temperature constant at 36.9°C by equalizing the heat gained and the heat lost by the body.

The body gains heat from

- the oxidation of food in the body tissues; heat production by this method is increased with bodily activity or exercise

- external sources such as the sun or heating appliances.

The body loses heat by

- the passage of heat from the skin to the surrounding air: the body is usually at a higher temperature than the air
- respiration: the air breathed out is usually warmer than the air breathed in
- the cooling effect of evaporation of perspiration from the surface of the skin: latent heat is taken from the skin to enable evaporation to take place. ·

Cooling effect of evaporation

To show the cooling effect of evaporation, surround the bulb of a 0°−100°C thermometer with cotton wool, holding it in position with thread or an elastic band. Note the temperature reading. Dip the cotton wool into ether and note the temperature as the ether evaporates, that is as it changes from liquid ether to ether vapour. To make this change, heat (known as **latent heat**) is required. The heat is taken from the surroundings—in this case the thermometer—and the reading is lowered. In the same way when perspiration evaporates, heat is taken from the skin resulting in the cooling of the body.

The body reacts automatically to moderate change in the surrounding conditions.

If the body becomes too hot

- Blood vessels in the skin are dilated, so increasing the amount of blood flowing near the surface of the body. This makes the skin red. Heat passes from the skin to the surrounding air.
- The production of perspiration is increased, leading to greater cooling of the skin by evaporation.

If the body becomes too cool

- Blood vessels are constricted so that less blood flows near the surface of the skin and less heat is lost to the surrounding air. The skin becomes white or blue.
- The secretion of perspiration is reduced.
- An attempt is made to trap an insulating layer of air between the body

hairs by contraction of the arrector pili muscles though this is ineffective due to lack of hair. The muscles are seen to be working as contraction pulls the skin into goose pimples as well as raising the hairs.

* Heat is produced by the muscular activity involved in shivering.

COMFORTABLE AIR CONDITIONS

Air conditions are affected by room temperature, humidity, and the movement and purity of the air.

Room temperature

The temperature in a salon should be kept constant at between 18°C and 20°C by regulation of heating appliances and ventilation. If the temperature is too low clients, particularly those with wet hair, will lose heat too quickly and feel cold. This will most probably occur early in the day if the salon has not been heated. The continual use of hair dryers and other heat-producing equipment tends to make the salon warmer as the day's work proceeds. As the room becomes warmer the rate of loss of heat from the surface of the skin decreases and the body may become uncomfortably warm. This factor is also affected by the type of clothing worn in the salon.

A wall thermometer is useful so that room temperature may be checked and heating and ventilation adjusted accordingly. The thermometer should be sited away from direct sunlight and other sources of heat such as radiators and hair dryers.

Humidity

If the humidity of the air is too low, the mucous membranes lining the nose and throat become uncomfortably dry and in this state they are easily infected. In the salon, however, the humidity tends to be high due to

* steam from the use of steamers and from hot water used during shampooing
* evaporation of water during the drying of hair
* moisture produced from the breath of people in the salon (air breathed out contains more moisture than air breathed in)
* evaporation of perspiration from the people in the salon.

If the air is too humid, evaporation of perspiration is prevented and the skin's cooling mechanism cannot work effectively. This results in the body overheating, and causes people to feel hot, tired and irritable, possibly leading to fainting. Good ventilation is required to control humidity.

Condensation

Excessive humidity may lead to problems of condensation. As warm moist air cools, it cannot hold as much moisture and the air may become saturated. If further cooling takes place, some of the moisture is deposited as liquid droplets as condensation takes place. This usually occurs if warm moist air comes into contact with cold surfaces such as a cold wall or window, a mirror or cold water pipes. Water is deposited on the surface, causing windows and mirrors to steam up, and droplets of water to trickle down the walls.

Condensation may be prevented if water vapour is continuously removed by good ventilation and the various surfaces such as walls and cold water pipes are insulated. Heaters may be placed alongside windows or the windows double glazed.

Hygrometer

A wall hygrometer may be used to measure humidity so that ventilation can be adjusted accordingly. A suitable hair hygrometer is shown in Fig. 2.1. The working of a hair hygrometer depends on the fact that hair is hygroscopic and increases in length as it absorbs moisture, decreasing in length if it loses moisture. The hygrometer contains a bundle of degreased hairs fixed at one end, with the other end attached through a spring to a pointer which moves over a scale.

As the humidity increases, the hairs absorb moisture, become longer and the spring pulls the pointer higher up the scale. If the humidity decreases, the hairs give up water to the air, become shorter and the spring moves the pointer lower on the scale. The hygrometer measures the humidity as a percentage.

$$\% \text{ Relative humidity} = \frac{\text{Actual weight of water vapour in any volume of air}}{\text{Weight of water vapour the air could hold, in the same volume at the same temperature}} \times 100$$

The relative humidity should be 50−70 per cent to ensure comfort.

Air movement

If the air in a salon is too still, increased local humidity close to the body prevents efficient evaporation of perspiration, leading to overheating.

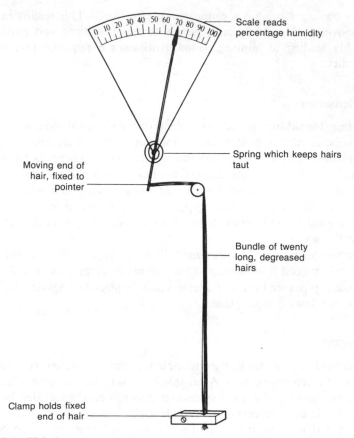

Fig. 2.1 Hair hygrometer

A variable speed fan is sometimes useful to keep the air moving in hot weather. If air is moving too quickly it may cause draughts which have a cooling effect. Good ventilation ensures fresh air without causing a draught.

Air purity

Frequent changes of salon air by good ventilation are necessary to remove pollutants affecting the purity of the air. These pollutants include:

- **Carbon dioxide**: during breathing, oxygen is used from the air and an increased amount of carbon dioxide is breathed out, though the effect of this is slight even in a badly ventilated room.
- **Excess moisture** causes high humidity.
- **Disease-causing micro-organisms**: viruses, causing infections such

as colds or 'flu, may be present in airborne droplets of moisture from the nose and mouth due to coughing, sneezing or even talking. Airborne dust, including particles of hair and scales of dead skin, may carry harmful bacteria.

- **Fumes** from chemicals used in the salon: gases, including unpleasant smells, quickly spread to all parts of the salon. Fumes from perm lotions, ammonia and hair spray may irritate the lining of the nose, throat or lungs.

SELF TESTING

1. What is normal body temperature (in degrees Celsius)?
2. How does the body increase heat loss if it is becoming overheated?
3. What is a suitable room temperature for a salon?
4. What is meant by humidity?
5. What are the sources of humidity in a salon?
6. How can humidity be measured?
7. For what reason may salon mirrors 'steam up'?
8. What is the effect of lack of movement of the air in a salon?
9. What pollutants may cause loss of purity of the air in a salon?

HEATING APPLIANCES

How heat travels

There are three ways in which heat can pass from one point to another: conduction, convection and radiation.

Conduction

Conduction from molecule to molecule through a solid can be illustrated by attaching several drawing pins to a metal rod by means of melted wax and, when the wax has solidified, supporting the rod (as shown in Fig. 2.2). On heating the unsupported end of the rod in a bunsen flame the pins drop off the rod in turn, proving that the heat is being gradually passed along the bar.

Convection

Convection takes place through a liquid or a gas by movement of hot particles. The stream of moving heated particles is called a **convection current**. Convection can be demonstrated in water by use of potassium

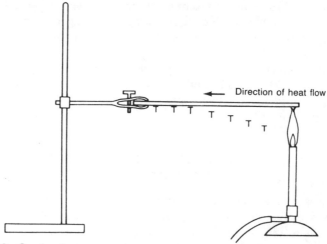

Fig. 2.2   Conduction

permanganate crystals, which give a purple colour to the moving particles (Fig. 2.3). Convection in air can be demonstrated by use of the apparatus shown in Fig. 2.4. The air heated by the candle flame rises and sets up a convection current of moving smoke.

Radiation

Radiation is in the form of rays or waves which travel in straight lines, such as heat from the sun or from a hot element in an electric fire (see Fig. 2.8b).

Choosing a heating appliance

Most heating appliances make use of either convection or radiation but sometimes use both. The type of heating appliance suitable for a particular salon depends on the size and position of the salon and on the cost and availability of various fuels. Central heating systems which also supply hot water for salon use are common. Smaller salons may find it more economical to use small fixed heaters or occasionally portable appliances.

Heating systems work more efficiently if heat losses from the salon are reduced by insulation of floors by carpeting including the use of an underlay, installation of double glazing to windows, insulation of the roof space by fibre glass, cavity wall insulation, and well-fitting external doors which exclude draughts. Good ventilation should work along with heating to ensure the required temperature of 18°−21°C and maintain pleasant working conditions.

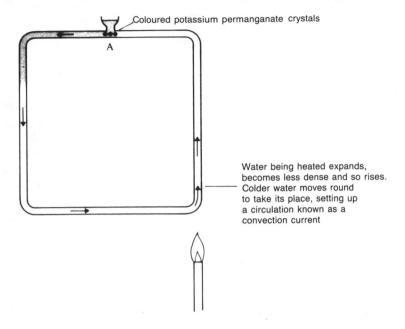

Fig. 2.3 Convection currents in a liquid

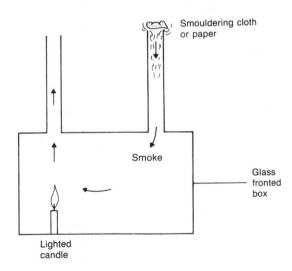

Fig. 2.4 Convection currents in a gas

Central heating systems

There are three main forms of central heating systems.

Circulation of hot water

Hot water from a boiler is circulated through narrow bore pipes by an electric pump to radiators, which give out heat to the room (see Fig. 2.5). The term 'radiator' implies transfer of heat by radiation, though most of the heat is transferred to the air and circulates in the rooms by convection. The operating temperature may be controlled by a wall thermostat or a separate thermostat on each radiator. The boiler may also be controlled by a time switch. This type of installation usually provides a supply of hot water for the salon as well. The radiators require wall space, which may present difficulties in a salon where much of the equipment is wall based.

Ducted warm air

Warm air is circulated through ducts by fans, and enters rooms by grilles near the floor (see Fig. 2.6). The electrical system is similar to a large fan-controlled storage heater and uses off-peak electricity. Heat travels round the rooms by convection of hot air.

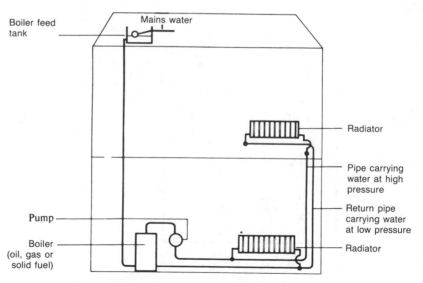

Fig. 2.5 Central heating by hot water

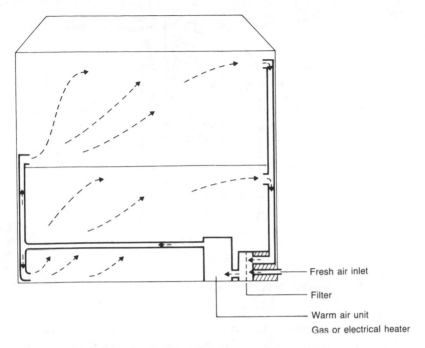

Fresh air inlet

Filter

Warm air unit
Gas or electrical heater

Fig. 2.6   Central heating by ducted warm air

Floor warming

In new buildings, an under-floor electrical heating system may be installed using off-peak electricity during the night. Heating elements are embedded in concrete floors and are thermostatically controlled. Hairdressers are standing all day and they may find this type of heating tiring to the feet.

Other fixed heaters

There are three main types of fixed heaters.

Gas convector heaters with a balanced flue

Gas convector heaters are safe for salon use as the flames are entirely enclosed (see **Fig. 2.7**). They are usually connected through an outside wall using a balanced flue. The combustion chamber of the heater is then completely isolated and sealed so that the gases produced during combustion cannot enter the room. Combined radiant and convector gas

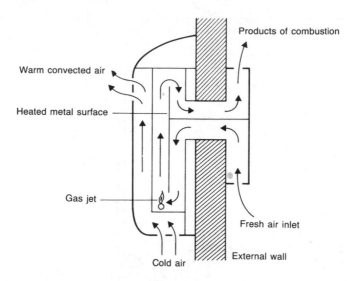

Fig. 2.7 Gas convector heater with a balanced flue

heaters are also available, the radiant elements providing quick warmth and a pleasant glow. They do, however, present a fire risk in a salon and are not normally recommended. All gas appliances require regular servicing to ensure safety.

Wall-mounted radiant electrical heaters

This type of heater is safe for salon use, as it has a pull-cord switch and is usually mounted high on the wall (see Figs 2.8a and 2.8b). The heating element is enclosed in a silica sheath and the reflector behind the element is pivoted so that the heat can be directed as required.

Electric storage heaters

The heating elements are embedded in heat-retaining bricks and heating takes place at night using off-peak electricity (see Figs 2.9a and 2.9b). Heat stored in the bricks is given out gradually during the following day. Greater control of the heat output is possible if the heaters are fan assisted.

Portable heaters

Portable heaters may be useful to provide local heating of a particular area though they may present a risk due to trailing flexes. Radiant electric

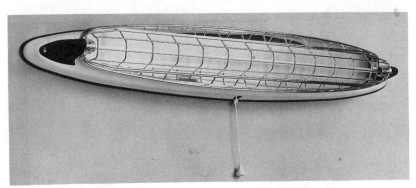

Fig. 2.8a Wall mounted radiant heater

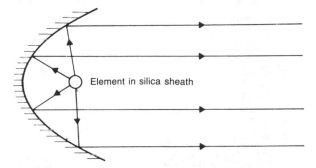

Element in silica sheath

Fig. 2.8b Reflection of radiant heat

fires, although always fitted with a guard, are not recommended as they present a risk if people stand too close. The three types of heaters listed here as portable are also available as fixed wall-mounted appliances and are safer in that form.

Oil-filled radiators

An electrical heating element in the base of the radiator creates a circulation of hot oil within the radiator. Heat is also transferred to the room by convection. The heaters are safe for salon use as there is no visible element. They are expensive to run and are usually fitted with a time switch and a thermostat.

Fan heaters

These work by forced convection in the same way as a hair dryer. An electric motor turns a fan which blows cool air over a heating element (see Figs 2.10a and 2.10b).

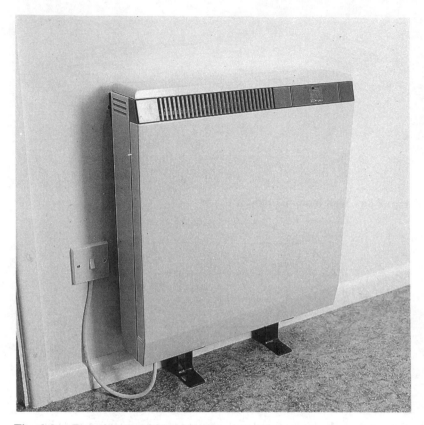

Fig. 2.9a Electric storage heater

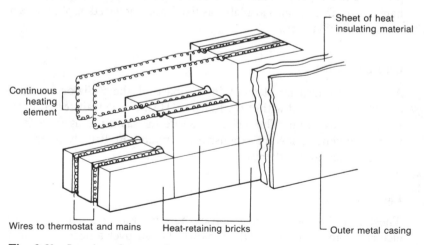

Sheet of heat insulating material

Continuous heating element

Wires to thermostat and mains   Heat-retaining bricks   Outer metal casing

Fig. 2.9b Interior of storage heater

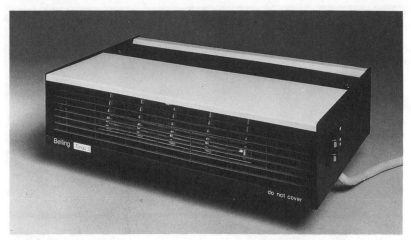

Fig. 2.10a Fan heater

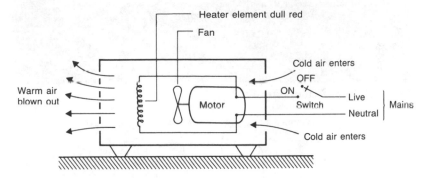

Fig. 2.10b Working diagram

Convector heaters

Convectors give a good background heat and are safe for salon use as there is no visible element. Convection currents are set up as the air circulates through the appliance (see Figs 2.11a and 2.11b).

SALON VENTILATION

Good ventilation should replace stale air with fresh air without causing a draught. To ensure this the following conditions should be satisfied:

• The air in the salon should be changed three or four times an hour.

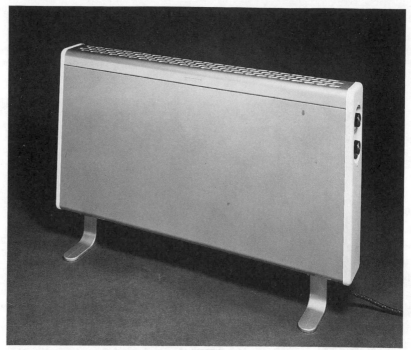

Fig. 2.11a Convector heater

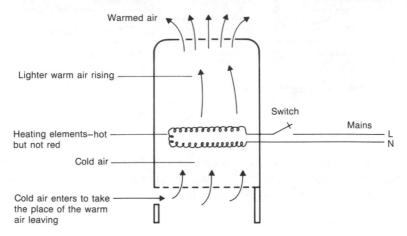

Fig. 2.11b Working diagram

- Cool air should not enter the room at floor level as this is draughty to the feet.
- Air entering the room above head level should be directed upwards so that it is slightly warmed before moving downwards. Clients with

wet hair feel a cooling effect due to the evaporation of moisture, and
further cooling by a down draught of cool air could be unpleasant.
- Air outlets should be smaller than inlets so that air does not circulate
too quickly.

Methods of ventilation

A salon may be ventilated by natural or artificial means.

Natural ventilation

Natural ventilation includes the use of windows, doors and ventilating
bricks. This type of ventilation depends on convection currents, and may
be assisted by the heating appliances in the salon.

The warm air of the salon, being less dense than the cold air, rises
and may pass out of the room through open windows high on the outside
walls or through ventilation bricks. Fresh air enters by windows and
doors, though its entry is difficult to control. Draughts may be caused,
blowing cut hair about. Dust, smoke or fumes from passing traffic may
blow into the salon. Some control is possible by fitting **Cooper's discs**
in windows. The inner disc can be rotated so that its openings coincide
with similar holes in the window (see Fig. 2.12).

Hopper windows make good inlets as they direct the air upwards on
entry (see Fig. 2.13).

Louvred windows consist of movable strips of glass (see Fig. 2.14).

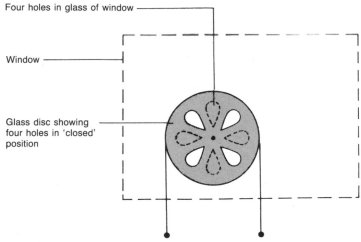

Four holes in glass of window

Window

Glass disc showing
four holes in 'closed'
position

Fig. 2.12 Cooper's disc

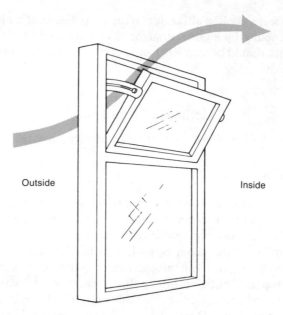

Outside

Inside

Fig. 2.13 Hopper window

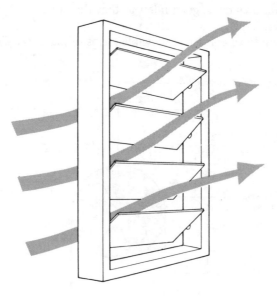

Fig. 2.14 Louvred window

They may be used as outlets or inlets of air according to the position of the strips when the louvres are open.

Artificial ventilation

Artificial or assisted ventilation involves the use of mechanical aids. This type of ventilation is more easily controlled than natural ventilation and is much more efficient.

Extractor fans are the simplest and most popular means of ventilation for a small salon. The fans are operated by an electric motor and are normally fitted into windows or outside walls. There are various sizes, with different speeds of action, and some can be switched to air intake as well as extraction. Extractor fans should not be sited near inlets because fresh air would be extracted immediately on entering, leaving stale air in the salon (see Fig. 2.15). To ensure full circulation the fan should be placed high up in the wall or window furthest from the door or other inlet. If the salon is small with no suitable outer wall, extractor fans may be fitted to inner walls or ceilings and the stale air carried outside by ducting.

The number or size of fans can be calculated from manufacturer's data, room size and the number of changes of air required per hour.

Example: Room size = 8 m × 4 m × 3 m = 96 m^3 (cubic metres)
Number of air changes required = 4 per hour
Therefore, air movement = 96 × 4 = 384 m^3 per hour.

A fan removing air at this rate may be chosen from the manufacturer's data.

In large buildings, an **exhaust system** using powerful extractor fans in the roof may withdraw stale air through ducts, and fresh air enters through windows and doors. Alternatively, in the **plenum system**, fresh air is forced into the building by fans, so increasing the air pressure inside

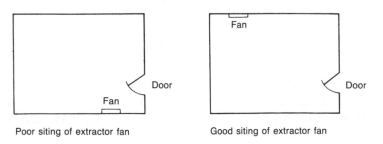

Poor siting of extractor fan   Good siting of extractor fan

Fig. 2.15 Siting an extractor fan

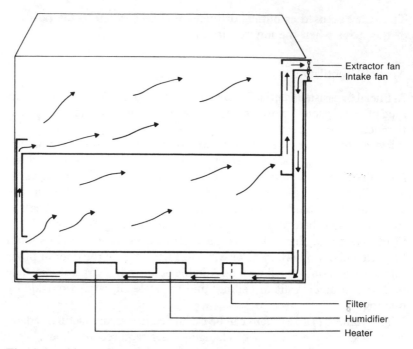

Fig. 2.16   Air conditioning of a building

and preventing incoming draughts. Any air leakage consists of stale air passing outwards through windows and doors.

The plenum and exhaust system may be combined to form a **balanced system** in which both intake of fresh air and extraction of stale air are controlled by fans in the roof. A more complicated balanced system in which air is filtered and adjusted to a suitable temperature and humidity is known as **air conditioning** (see Fig. 2.16). Small air conditioning units are available to control the air in a single room. These sometimes recirculate the air after filtering and adjusting the temperature.

SELF TESTING

1. State three ways in which heat can pass from one point to another.
2. What is meant by a convection current?
3. How would under-floor heating affect the comfort of a hairdresser?
4. Why is a flue necessary for gas heaters?
5. What is the purpose of ventilation?
6. Why should air, entering a room at above head level, be directed upwards?

7. For maximum efficiency where should extractor fans be sited in a salon?
8. What is meant by 'natural ventilation'?
9. Why may natural ventilation be inefficient and what can be done to improve its efficiency?
10. What types of artificial ventilation are available?

SALON LIGHTING

The lighting for a salon should be, as far as possible, by natural daylight but when this is inadequate some form of artificial lighting is required.
Good artificial lighting should ensure the following:

- An even distribution of **well-diffused** (scattered) general lighting over the whole salon, so avoiding contrasting brightly lit and dark areas which may cause discomfort and eye strain when moving about the salon.
- Additional **localized** lighting where required in working areas, possibly over the reception desk and dressing tables.
- Particularly good lighting on **stairs**, with lights sited so that no shadows are cast over the treads.
- Avoidance of **glare** from bright unshaded lights or bright lights reflected through mirrors, causing discomfort and eye strain due to the bright light shining into the eyes. This involves the careful siting of both lights and mirrors.
- Artificial light with a colour as near as possible to that of **daylight** so avoiding difficulties when colouring hair. This will be considered again in Chapter 15 on Colouring Hair.

Sources of artificial light

Artificial light can be produced from tungsten filament lamps (ordinary electric light bulbs) or by fluorescent tubes.

Filament lamps

Filament lamps (see Fig. 2.17) give out light when the filament becomes white hot. They have low efficiency because a large amount of unwanted heat is produced as well as light. Clear glass bulbs cast sharp shadows and, if unshaded, may cause glare due to the brightness of the filament. Pearl bulbs, which are frosted on the inside, and opal bulbs, which have an internal white coating, prevent glare by concealing the filament.

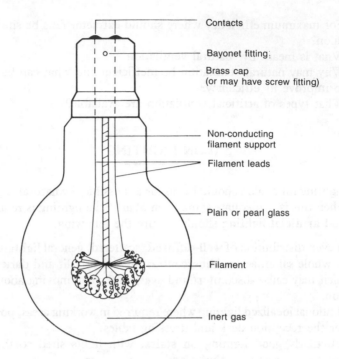

Fig. 2.17   Tungsten filament lamp

Internally silvered bulbs reflect light from a silvered surface to produce a narrow beam used in spotlighting.

Filament bulbs give a reddish-yellow light with less blue than daylight. This makes colour matching difficult. Blue and green shades appear darker and red shades brighter than in daylight.

Fluorescent tubes

In fluorescent tubes (see Fig. 2.18), an electric current is conducted through mercury vapour and this produces ultra-violet light. The inside of the tube is coated with a fluorescent powder called a **phosphor** which converts the ultra-violet light into ordinary visible light. The colour of the light produced varies from a bluish white to a warm white according to the type of phosphor used. White fluorescent lighting has less red and yellow than daylight so makes blue and green pigments look brighter and red shades darker. **Warm white** tubes give a light similar to daylight and are to be preferred for salon use. Fluorescent lighting of this type is thus more suitable for hair-colouring work than that from filament lamps. The tubes give a soft diffused light free from glare and casting very little shadow.

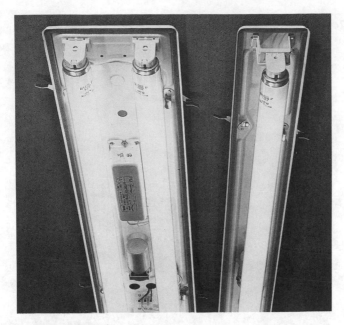

Fig. 2.18 Fluorescent tubes

Straight fluorescent tubes are available in various lengths, or the tubes may be shaped into a more compact form designed to take the place of a filament lamp. These miniature fluorescent lamps may be installed in special fittings or adapted for the lampholders previously suitable only for filament lamps (see Fig. 2.19).

Fluorescent lamps are more efficient than filament lamps because they give out very little heat. They are therefore cheaper to run and also have a longer life than filament bulbs, though they are more expensive to buy. The cool running of fluorescent tubes makes them particularly suitable for salons, especially where artificial light is used throughout the day and where overheating of the salon may become a problem.

General purpose light fittings

General purpose lighting is designed to give a uniform illumination over the whole salon; it may be achieved by several methods.

Diffused illumination

General diffused illumination is produced when a filament lamp is enclosed in a translucent glass or plastic globe which diffuses the light

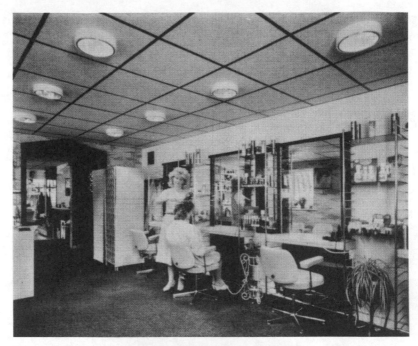

Fig. 2.19a   Salon lit by miniature fluorescent bulbs

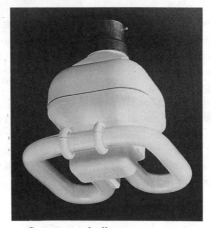

Fig. 2.19b   Miniature fluorescent bulb

as it passes through the shade (see Fig. 2.20), or when a fluorescent tube is enclosed in an opal plastic diffuser (see Fig. 2.21).

Indirect illumination

Indirect illumination results from a filament lamp concealed by an opaque fitting directing the light upwards to the ceiling. Reflection from the

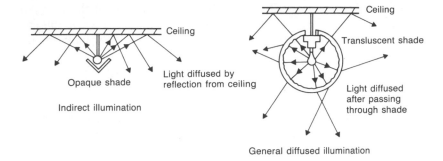

Ceiling

Opaque shade

Light diffused by
reflection from ceiling

Indirect illumination

Ceiling

Transluscent shade

Light diffused
after passing
through shade

General diffused illumination

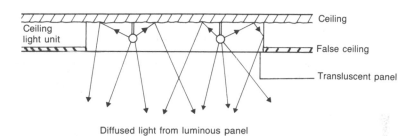

Ceiling
light unit

Ceiling

False ceiling

Transluscent panel

Diffused light from luminous panel

Fig. 2.20   General purpose lighting

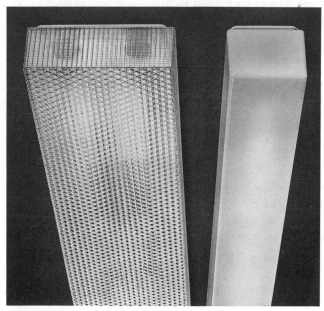

Fig. 2.21   (Left) Prismatic controller used to direct light downwards
(Right) Opal diffuser used to scatter light in all directions

ceiling diffuses and distributes the light rays over the whole salon (see Fig. 2.20). The colour of the ceiling is particularly important in this case and should preferably be white so as to reflect the maximum amount of light.

Luminous panels

Luminous panels concealing either filament lamps or fluorescent tubes behind sheets of translucent glass or plastic may be housed in a false ceiling (see Fig. 2.20). The whole ceiling acts as the source of illumination and a pleasantly diffused light is distributed over the room.

Localized light fittings

Localized lighting is designed to concentrate light on a small area such as a working surface or a special display.

Direct illumination

Direct illumination from a light fitting with a reflective shade is arranged to direct about 90 per cent of the light downwards (see Fig. 2.22b). **Spotlight bulbs** also give direct illumination and when fitted to a track may be angled and positioned to illuminate special displays or pictures (see Figs 2.22a and 2.22b).

Plastic prismatic controllers

Fluorescent tubes may be fitted with clear plastic prismatic controllers containing a series of prisms which direct the light downwards in a chosen direction (see Fig. 2.21).

Safety notes

- Replace damaged light fittings immediately to avoid electric shock.
- Switch off the electricity supply before replacing light bulbs.
- Replace flickering fluorescent tubes as they may affect people who are subject to migraine or epilepsy.

SELF TESTING

1. What are the requirements for good artificial lighting in a salon?

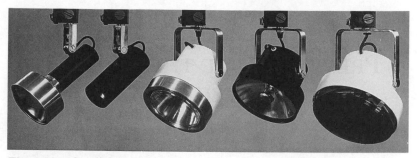

Fig. 2.22a   Spotlights

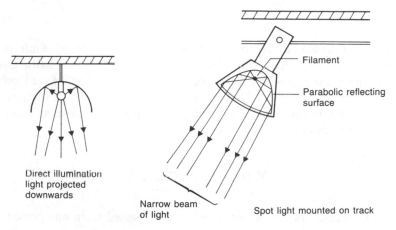

Direct illumination
light projected
downwards

Narrow beam
of light

Filament

Parabolic reflecting
surface

Spot light mounted on track

Fig. 2.22b   Localized lighting

2. What is meant by diffused lighting?
3. What is meant by 'glare'?
4. What are the causes of glare?
5. How can glare be avoided?
6. Why are filament lamps less efficient than fluorescent tubes?
7. Why are 'warm white' fluorescent tubes recommended for salon use?
8. Which types of light fittings are designed to give uniform lighting over the whole salon?
9. What is meant by indirect illumination?

3
PREVENTION OF THE SPREAD OF INFECTION

Hairdressers have a duty to their clients to prevent the spread of infection in the salon as far as possible. The close contact between the hairdresser and client, the ease with which infections can be spread by infected tools, and the warm moist air of a salon provide ideal conditions for the spread of infection unless special attention is given to personal and salon hygiene, the sterilization of tools and salon ventilation.

WHAT IS INFECTION?

An infectious disease is one which can be passed from one person to another. Infection itself is caused by the presence of **micro-organisms** which may be classified as fungi, bacteria and viruses. Though there are many differences between them, disease-causing bacteria and viruses are together commonly known as 'germs'. Germs can cause infection when they enter the body through breaks in the skin, by being breathed in, or through the mouth.

Fungi

Fungi tend to grow on the outside of the body, the commonest fungal infections being various forms of **ringworm** including ringworm of the skin, scalp, nails, beard and feet (athlete's foot). The fungus grows into a mass of long thread-like cells called a **mycelium** (see Figs 3.1a and 3.1b). The threads pierce the surface of the skin and can grow into the hair shafts, so weakening the hair. They secrete a digestive juice which breaks down keratin, the main protein of skin and hair, to provide the fungus with nourishment. The spread of fungal diseases takes place when portions of the mycelium break away and are carried on to the skin or

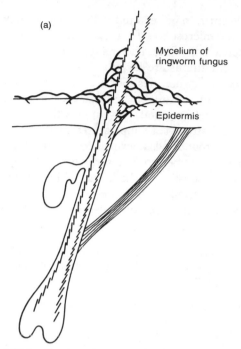

Fig. 3.1a Hair follicle showing ringworm fungus

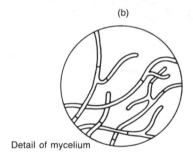

Fig. 3.1b Detail of mycelium

hair of another person. Treatment of fungal diseases of the skin is by a drug, terbinafine which is taken orally.

Bacteria

Bacteria are present almost everywhere around us, in the air, in soil, in water, and on most surfaces including the surface of the skin. Some bacteria cause disease and are called **pathogens**, but many are harmless.

Bacteria are too small to be seen individually by the naked eye but may be seen through a microscope. Each bacterium consists of a single cell, which is a complete unit of life. Bacteria reproduce themselves by splitting into two and if conditions are favourable reproduction may take place as often as every twenty minutes. For growth and reproduction, bacteria require food, moisture, a suitable temperature and usually oxygen. Low temperatures, as in refrigeration, prevent growth but do not kill bacteria. Most bacteria are destroyed at temperatures above 70°C. Those affecting the skin are usually round cells known as cocci. **Streptococci** are arranged in chains and cause impetigo and sore throats. **Staphylococci** form bunches and are responsible for boils and folliculitis though often both types of cocci are present on the same site (see Fig. 3.2).

Bacterial infections may be controlled in the following ways:

On objects, such as hairdressing tools, they may be destroyed by

- chemical disinfectants, e.g. glutaraldehyde or cetrimide
- ultra-violet rays, e.g. in salon 'sterilizing' cabinets
- heating to about 70°C.

On the surface of the skin they may be controlled by

- antiseptics, e.g. cetrimide
- antibiotic ointments.

Inside the body they are treated by taking antibiotics orally or by injection, e.g. penicillin.

Viruses

Viruses (see Fig. 3.3) are smaller than bacteria but can be seen by using a powerful electron microscope. Viruses cause diseases such as colds, influenza and measles if they enter the body through the nose or mouth, and conditions such as simple herpes (cold sores) and warts if they enter breaks in the skin. Viruses multiply in the body cells, eventually destroying the cells in which they are living and liberating the viruses to attack other cells. Viruses do not live long once outside the human body but may be carried into the air in **droplets** from the nose or mouth during coughing and sneezing, so passing the infection to others. Virus diseases are, in general, more difficult to treat than bacterial diseases. **Antibodies** in the blood destroy viruses in the body. Two serious viral diseases of which hairdressers should be aware are AIDS and hepatitis B. These will be considered separately later in this chapter.

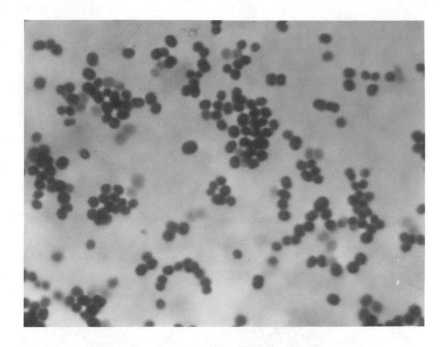

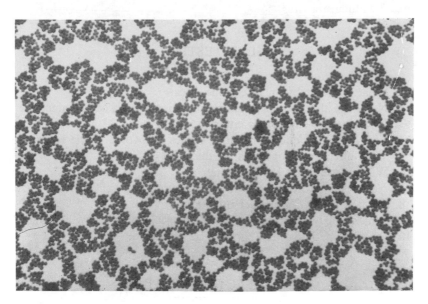

Fig. 3.2 Bacteria (a) streptococci (b) staphylococci

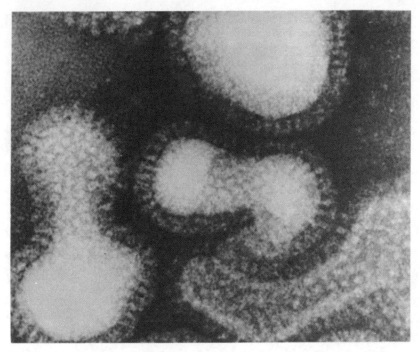

Fig. 3.3 Influenza virus

SELF TESTING

1. What is meant by an infectious disease?
2. Name the three kinds of micro-organism which cause infection.
3. In what ways can germs enter the body?
4. Which kind of micro-organism causes ringworm of the scalp?
5. What effect has ringworm on the hair?
6. What is meant by a pathogen?
7. Name two infections caused by bacteria.
8. What is meant by droplet infection?
9. Which kind of micro-organism is responsible for the growth of warts?
10. By what methods may bacteria be destroyed?

HOW INFECTION IS SPREAD

In a salon, infection may be spread from one person to another by direct and indirect contact.

Direct contact

Direct contact with the infected person can lead to droplet infection through inhaling airborne droplets coming from the nose or mouth of an infected person while coughing, sneezing or speaking. Colds, influenza and measles may be spread in this way. Infection can result from touching an infected area of a person's body. Ringworm, impetigo and boils may be spread by touch. Infections which are spread by touch are said to be **contagious**. Infection can be caused by contact with infected blood if it enters breaks in the skin.

Indirect contact

Indirect contact through the use of an infected tool or contact with infected hair or towels involves **cross-infection**, which is the passing of infection from a person to an object and the subsequent transfer of that infection from the object to a second person. The two people involved may never actually meet and could have entered the salon on different occasions. Ringworm fungus may be transmitted via hair brushes, and impetigo through infected towels.

CONTROL OF INFECTION

Airborne infections such as colds, 'flu, etc, can be minimized by avoiding contact with infected people and by good ventilation.

* Hairdressers with very heavy colds or 'flu should stay at home.
* If clients have heavy colds make sure salon ventilation is good.

The spread of **skin infections** can largely be controlled by making sure that areas of broken skin are covered to prevent the entry of germs, by the efficient sterilization of tools, and by attention to the cleanliness of the salon.

* Tools should be washed, adequately disinfected, and kept in a clean place before use on a client.
* Ideally each hairdresser should have two sets of tools to allow time for full sterilization of tools between clients if necessary.
* During use, tools should be placed on a clean paper towel on the dressing table and never placed in an overall pocket. Hair pins and clips must not be held in the mouth.
* Any tool dropped on to the floor should be washed and disinfected before re-use.

- Each client requires clean towels. Drying towels without first washing them is unhygienic, as germs will multiply in the warmth during drying.
- All soiled towels should be kept in a covered bin. They should be machine washed at the highest possible temperature (95°C).
- Clients with minor skin infections, such as boils, may be treated normally but care should be taken not to touch the area and tools should be sterilized after use. Disposable neck-strips may be useful.
- Clients with more serious infections, such as ringworm, should not be offered any salon services. It must be tactfully suggested that they consult a doctor. Where the condition is unnoticed until work has begun, complete the service as briefly as possible. Tools which have been used should be sterilized by autoclave if possible. Towels and gowns should be washed immediately. All hair trimmings should be burned.
- Always avoid contact with blood from a client.
- Cuts and abrasions on a hairdresser's hands must be kept covered.
- A hairdresser's hands should be washed before and after attending to a client, after every use of the toilet, and after blowing the nose. Hands should be dried using a paper towel.

AIDS (ACQUIRED IMMUNE DEFICIENCY SYNDROME)

AIDS is a serious viral infection caused by a virus known as HIV (Human Immunodeficiency Virus). At present there is no cure for AIDS. The virus attacks cells in the blood which normally produce the antibodies required to fight infection. A person may be a carrier of the virus for many years without becoming ill and there are no means of telling whether or not a healthy-looking client is a carrier of the AIDS virus. There is no danger from a carrier while the skin remains intact. A risk occurs only if a client who has the AIDS virus bleeds as a result of a cut or scratch, and the client's blood enters a cut or other break in the hairdresser's skin (e.g. an inflamed area of dermatitis). The possibility of infection with the AIDS virus by this method is very slight indeed. However, contact with a client's blood must be avoided and any blood inadvertently coming into contact with the hands should be washed off immediately. There is no danger of infection if cuts and abrasions on a hairdresser's hands are kept covered.

If a client's skin is accidentally cut or the skin punctured, the client should be asked to apply pressure to the cut or apply a pre-packed spirit swab. Though the AIDS virus has a very short life outside the body, any tool contaminated with blood should be immediately washed and sterilized before re-use.

In the unlikely event of a larger quantity of blood being shed, pour household bleach (sodium hypochlorite) over the area, leave for two to three minutes then, wearing disposable gloves, clean it away using a disposable cloth. Bleach is suitable for use on vinyl and tiled surfaces. Carpets and cloth fabrics, which are damaged by bleach, should be washed with detergent and hot water. Again, wear disposable gloves and use a disposable cloth.

HEPATITIS B

Hepatitis B is a serious viral infection which affects the liver. Like AIDS it can be transmitted by infected blood. The precautions used against AIDS will also serve as protection against hepatitis.

SELF TESTING

1. In what ways is infection spread by direct contact?
2. What is meant by a contagious disease?
3. What is meant by cross-infection?
4. By what methods could ringworm fungus be passed from person to person?
5. What steps would you take if you suspected that a client had ringworm of the scalp?
6. How can airborne infection be reduced in a salon?
7. Why should cuts and abrasions on a hairdresser's hands be kept covered?
8. Why should you avoid getting a client's blood on your skin?

TREATMENT OF TOOLS

Sterilization means the complete destruction of all living organisms on an object. This can rarely be achieved in a salon except by the use of moist heat in an autoclave, or by dry heat using high temperatures for an adequate period of time. **Disinfection** by liquid chemicals is more usual and will kill most germs if correctly carried out, but will not necessarily completely sterilize tools. Salon tools must always be washed before being sterilized or disinfected. **Antiseptics** are intended only for use on the skin to prevent wounds from becoming septic and are not used on tools. Prepared swabs impregnated with alcohol are useful for the treatment of minor wounds. Sterilized and disinfected tools may be stored in **ultra-violet cabinets**.

Sterilization

Moist heat

Boiling water or steam treatment will not sterilize tools unless accompanied by increased pressure as in the **autoclave**. This works on the same principle as a domestic pressure cooker (see Fig. 3.4). If water vapour is not allowed to escape from the container in which water is being heated, the pressure on the surface of the water is increased. This makes it more difficult for the molecules to leave the water until they are given more energy by raising the temperature. Thus increasing the pressure raises the boiling point of water. At normal atmospheric pressure, water boils at 100°C but on doubling the pressure the boiling point rises to about 120°C. Autoclaving is suitable for metal tools, glass, and rubber objects as well as some plastics. Electrically controlled automatic autoclaves are available and should be used according to the manufacturer's instructions. The process of sterilization takes about 15 minutes at a temperature of around 120°C.

Immediate autoclaving is essential for tools such as scissors and crochet hooks if they have pierced the skin of either a client or a hairdresser. This avoids the possible transfer of infected blood to the bloodstream of a second person. Such contaminated tools must not be used again before sterilization. They should be placed on a paper towel until treated by autoclaving and the towel immediately burned or enclosed in a plastic bag and sealed before disposal. Crochet hooks and the removable blades

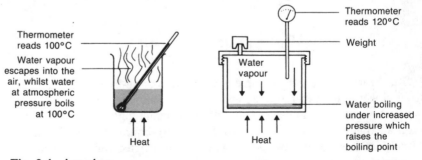

Fig. 3.4 Autoclave

of clippers should be autoclaved regularly. Scissors may be blunted during autoclaving and, unless they have penetrated the skin, are normally washed in detergent and water then dried, or wiped with a prepared alcohol wipe and left to dry.

Dry heat

Glass bead sterilizers using dry heat may be used instead of an autoclave but need 30 minutes to heat before sterilization can commence, will generally take only one long instrument at once, are unsuitable for such items as clipper blades and, as they work at higher temperatures, tend to blunt or damage tools more. They should be used according to the manufacturer's instructions because the time required for sterilization depends on the temperature attained.

Naked flames may be used to treat small metal tools but blunting may occur and the method has little practical value in hairdressing.

Burning destroys pathogens: salon rubbish such as cut hair and infected tissues may be disposed of by this method.

Disinfection

Liquid chemical disinfectants will kill germs if used long enough and strong enough and may be effectively used to reduce the risk of infection in salons. Suitable disinfectants include the following.

Glutaraldehyde

Glutaraldehyde (e.g. Cidex) is used in a 2 per cent solution in a covered container to soak metal tools and has replaced the use of formaldehyde, which was formerly used in salon sterilizing cabinets. The use of glutaraldehyde is the best method of disinfection of tools if an autoclave is not available. The solution remains effective for about 14 days, after which it must be discarded. It must be used with care. Wear protective gloves to avoid allergic reaction. Avoid inhaling the vapour and keep the container covered. Rinse tools before use on the skin.

Quaternary ammonium compounds

Quaternary ammonium compounds (e.g. cetrimide) are often used in a 1–2 per cent solution in a disinfectant jar on dressing out tables to hold combs between use on clients. The solution should be changed regularly to remain effective.

Alcohol

Alcohol (70 per cent alcohol or surgical spirit) or alcohol with chlorhexidene is used as a wipe for clipper blades, scissors, and the heads of crimping irons, curling tongs, and so on.

Hypochlorites

Hypochlorites (household bleaches) are used mostly for cleaning purposes and treatment of blood spills.

Ultra-violet cabinets

Ultra-violet cabinets are used in many salons. Ultra-violet rays are produced by a mercury vapour lamp sited at the top of the cabinet. The rays have disinfectant properties but as rays travel only in straight lines, objects must be turned frequently to expose all surfaces to the radiation. Objects should be grease-free as the rays are absorbed by grease. The recommended exposure time is 20 minutes for each surface. This type of cabinet is best used for storing equipment which has previously been sterilized by autoclave or disinfected by chemical methods. Ultra-violet rays are damaging to the eyes and skin, therefore the lamp switches off automatically as the door opens.

SALON CLEANLINESS

Along with personal hygiene and the cleanliness of tools, the cleanliness of the salon itself is important in preventing the spread of infection. Surfaces such as dressing tables, basins, walls, floors and chairs must be cleaned regularly by washing with hot water and detergent. Cupboards and shelves where instruments, towels and gowns are stored must have smooth surfaces free from crevices which may harbour germs.

Inorganic dust may originate from the ash of cigarettes or particles of grit from roads. **Organic dust** may consist of flakes of dead skin, small pieces of hair or fluff from clothing and towels. Dust mixed with moisture or grease forms **dirt.** This is best removed by use of a detergent and hot water with an abrasive powder to break up the dirt if necessary.

Cut hair should be swept up immediately and placed in a plastic bag in a covered bin along with waste cotton wool and soiled paper towels. Waste bags should be sealed or tied before removal from the salon each night and disposed of through the normal refuse collection or if possible burned.

SELF TESTING

1. What is the difference between sterilization and disinfection?
2. Name two methods of sterilization.
3. What is the purpose of an antiseptic?
4. Why should scissors or crochet hooks be sterilized if they have pierced a client's skin?
5. How are scissors normally disinfected if they have not pierced the skin?
6. Name the chemical disinfectant often used to treat combs between use on clients.
7. What precautions should be taken in the use of glutaraldehyde?
8. What type of disinfectant is suitable for use on crimping irons?
9. What is the main use of an ultra-violet cabinet in a salon?
10. What is the correct way to deal with hair cuttings?

4

SAFETY AND FIRST AID

The legal requirements for safety in a salon are laid down in the **Health and Safety at Work Act 1974** and the updated **Workplace (Health, Safety and Welfare) Regulations 1992**. Under the Act **employers** are responsible for the provision of safe and well-maintained equipment, safe methods of use and storage of dangerous materials, the provision of fire exits, firefighting appliances and first aid equipment. They must also ensure that staff are trained in safety and health matters connected with their work, and these duties are extended to ensure the safety and welfare of members of the public entering the salon. **Employees** also have a duty under the Act to take reasonable care of the health and safety of both themselves and of persons who may be affected by their work.

The emphasis should be on the prevention of accidents but it is also essential to be able to deal efficiently with accidents if they do occur.

All members of staff should know

- how to telephone for an ambulance or the Fire Service
- how to use the salon fire extinguisher
- the position of the main stop tap for water
- the position of the main switch for electricity
- the basic first aid procedures and the position of the salon first aid box
- the whereabouts of a torch kept for emergency use in case the salon electricity supply is unexpectedly cut off.

PREVENTION OF ACCIDENTS

Accidents may involve falling, mistreatment of the client, electrical equipment, chemical substances, and fire.

Accidents involving falling

These may be minimized by ensuring the following:

- The salon is well lit, without any dark areas.
- The floor has a non-slip surface and is kept free from spilled substances on which people may slip.
- There are no trailing flexes to electrical appliances.
- Furniture and equipment have no dangerous projections.
- There are no obstructions over which people may fall, particularly in those areas where people normally walk.

Accidents involving mistreatment of the client

Accidents to clients should be prevented by the hairdresser, who should note the following.

- Cuts are most likely to occur when cutting hair near the lobes of the ears or when cutting neck hairs.
- Careless use of hair pins and roller pins may result in piercing the client's skin.
- Burns may occur when using blow dryers, infra-red heaters or if metal clips touch the client's scalp during use of a hood dryer.
- Scalds may occur by using excessively hot water in shampooing, during the use of steamers or when giving hot oil treatments.

Accidents involving electrical equipment

The **Electricity at Work Regulations 1990** require that all electrical appliances used in the workplace are tested for safety by a qualified electrician at least once a year, and that a written record of the tests is kept for inspection by the Health and Safety authorities. This should ensure that the appliances themselves are in good order, but correct usage is also important. The safety devices incorporated in all electrical circuits are described in Chapter 5.

Prevention of electrical accidents

Accidents resulting in electric shock may be avoided by

- replacing frayed flexes and damaged plugs and switches
- switching off at the mains before replacing main fuses
- switching off the light switch before replacing lamps

- disconnecting equipment for cleaning and examination for faults
- never handling electrical equipment with wet hands or while standing on a wet floor.

Accidents involving chemical substances

The **Control of Substances Hazardous to Health (COSHH) Act 1989** requires employers to assess the health risk of substances used at work. These include substances which are

- **corrosive** to the skin, e.g. sodium hydroxide used in hair straighteners or relaxers
- **irritants** which are not corrosive but which on repeated contact with the skin can cause inflammation, e.g. ammonium thioglycollate in perm lotions, para dyes (permanent hair dyes), and glutaraldehyde used to disinfect tools
- **harmful if inhaled**, e.g. lacquer fumes, powder bleach and dry powder shampoo.

Hazard warning symbols

Under the **Labelling of Dangerous Substances Regulations 1984**, manufacturers are required to place hazard warning symbols (see Fig. 4.1) on the containers of dangerous products. These include (besides the hazardous substances mentioned above)

- **gaseous and highly flammable substances**, e.g. propane, butane and alcohol in aerosol hair sprays and mousses
- **oxidizing substances**, e.g. hydrogen peroxide, which gives off oxygen gas when heated and so assists fire
- **toxic substances**.

Prevention of chemical accidents

Accidents with chemicals may usually be avoided by careful handling and by always following the manufacturer's instructions. In particular ensure that these precautions are taken:

- Protective gloves are worn for perming, permanent colouring and removal of tools from glutaraldehyde disinfectant.
- The inhalation of hair spray and powder bleaches is avoided.
- Chemicals do not run into the client's eyes or on to the skin.
- Chemicals are kept out of reach of children.
- All containers are clearly labelled. Liquids should be poured from

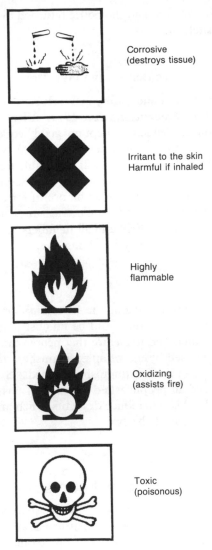

Corrosive
(destroys tissue)

Irritant to the skin
Harmful if inhaled

Highly
flammable

Oxidizing
(assists fire)

Toxic
(poisonous)

Fig. 4.1 Hazard symbols

the side of the bottle away from the label so that the label is not damaged by liquid running down the side of the bottle.
- Chemicals are never placed in bottles commonly used for lemonade, squash, etc.
- Quantities are accurately measured and not merely guessed.
- Once chemicals have been poured from storage bottles, any surplus is discarded and not poured back into the bottle.

- The stopper is replaced, and the bottle returned to its correct storage place immediately after use.

Accidents involving fire

In addition to the Health and Safety at Work Act, fire precautions are covered by the **Fire Precautions Act 1971**. All premises must have firefighting equipment which is kept in good working order and is suitable for the type of fire most likely to occur. A compressed carbon dioxide type extinguisher (see Fig. 4.2) is suitable for salon use, but it should be tested every three months by the Fire Service to maintain its efficiency. Sand or a fire blanket may be useful for dealing with small fires. Water must never be used on electrical fires or on burning oil. There should be regular fire drill and all members of staff should know how to deal with an emergency involving fire.

Dealing with fires

In the event of a fire in the salon, the first consideration must be the safety of the occupants. There should be no obstructions to exits, and doors must be left unlocked to ensure that people can leave quickly. A small fire can be tackled by use of an extinguisher, aiming the flow at the base of the fire. If it is not extinguished immediately, the Fire Service should be called and all people asked to leave. If possible all windows and doors should be closed to reduce draughts which may fan the flames, and to delay the spread of the fire.

Prevention of fire accidents

Fire risks may be decreased by the following precautions.

- Use flammable products such as aerosol lacquers and mousses with care. These products are a potential fire risk and should be stored in relatively small quantities. Hydrogen peroxide, which assists fire, should not be stored near flammable substances.
- Use electrical equipment properly. Avoid overloading circuits, use the correct size of fuse for each appliance (see Chapter 5) and examine equipment regularly to avoid faulty insulation and faulty appliances.
- Never drape towels over the vents of convector heaters or hair dryers while in use as this prevents the circulation of air, causing overheating of the appliance.
- Ensure that cigarette ends are completely extinguished and that ash

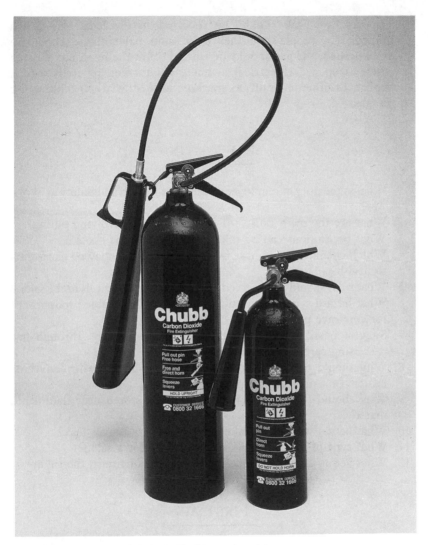

Fig. 4.2 Compressed carbon dioxide extinguisher

trays are provided. Smoking should, of course, be discouraged wherever possible.

- Avoid emptying ash trays into waste bins containing combustible material and make sure that all rubbish is removed from the building at the end of the day.
- Use gas appliances carefully. They should be regularly serviced to ensure correct working. Escaping gas can explode if ignited and any

suspected gas leak should be reported to the local Gas Board immediately. People should leave the salon, naked flames should be extinguished, the gas should be turned off at the main tap and the windows opened. Electrical switches should not be used to turn appliances either on or off, as sparking inside the switch could ignite the gas.

SELF TESTING

1. What is the duty of employees under the Health and Safety at Work Act?
2. What are the main causes of salon accidents involving falling?
3. What precautions can be taken to avoid electric shock?
4. Which chemical substances used in hairdressing may be hazardous to health?
5. What rules should be observed when handling chemicals in the salon?
6. What hazard symbol is used (a) for highly flammable products (b) for corrosive products?
7. Suggest possible ways in which a hairdresser may, through not exercising care, damage a client's skin.
8. Why should towels never be draped over air vents in convector heaters or hair dryers during use?
9. Why should hydrogen peroxide never be stored near flammable materials?
10. What action would you take if you suspected a gas leak?
11. What type of fire extinguisher is suitable for a salon?
12. What action should be taken in the event of fire in the salon?

FIRST AID

In cases of accident or illness in the salon, a hairdresser should be capable of rendering first aid. Regular clients may give information about their health during conversation and these comments should be mentally noted since it may be useful to know, in an emergency, that a client is a diabetic, has a heart condition or suffers from epilepsy. Such clients may also carry cards with instructions for treatment, and tablets or inhalants for emergency use. Most cases requiring attention in the salon will be minor accidents such as small cuts or slight burns. At the same time the hairdresser is responsible for the care and safety of clients and must deal with any emergency arising, however serious. It is important to stress the need for calling medical aid or an ambulance in good time if required, remembering also to pass on as much information as possible about the patient.

Bleeding

A first-aider should always keep any open cuts or wounds covered and avoid contact with blood from another person. Such blood should be washed off the first-aider's skin immediately. Blood spills should be disinfected by pouring household bleach over the area and leaving for two to three minutes before cleaning away, using a disposable cloth and a lot of water. Disposable gloves must always be worn when dealing with blood spills. In all cases of bleeding the aim of treatment is to prevent loss of blood and to avoid infection of the wound.

Cuts and small punctured wounds

Minor cuts on the back of the neck or lobe of the ear may be caused accidentally by scissors or razors, and small punctured wounds may result from the careless use of hair pins or roller pins. To check the bleeding apply a prepared spirit swab and leave it to dry. Do not get the client's blood on your own hands. Place the used swab in a plastic bag and seal before disposal. An aerosol styptic may be used but stick styptics should be avoided as they may lead to cross-infection. Cover the wound with an adhesive dressing if necessary.

Nose bleeding

Let the patient sit with the head bent slightly forwards to prevent blood from running down the throat which may cause vomiting. Ask the patient to pinch the nostrils together tightly for a few minutes until bleeding has stopped by the formation of a clot. The patient should avoid blowing the nose for some time afterwards so that the clot is not disturbed.

Burns and scalds

Burns and scalds result in intense pain with redness of the skin, blisters or in severe cases destruction of tissue.

Burns

Burns may be caused by contact with a flame or hot metal, by an electric current passing through the body, by friction with a fast-moving object or by chemicals such as strong hydrogen peroxide or sodium hydroxide.

Burns due to electric current are often deep, but extensive burning of the skin surface is usually more serious.

Wash caustic chemicals off the skin immediately by flooding the area with cold water from a running tap, and remove any contaminated clothing as quickly as possible to prevent further burning. Treat other types of burns or scalds by running cold water gently over them from the tap or immersing them in cold water for 5–10 minutes to reduce the pain. If blisters occur, do not break them but cover them with a sterile dressing and bandage lightly. In severe cases cover the whole area, including clothing, with a sterile dressing and remove the patient to hospital as soon as possible. At first the burnt skin and clothing will be sterile due to the effect of the heat, so avoid infection by covering it quickly and by not touching the area or breathing over it. Reassure the patient, give cold drinks and keep the patient warm while awaiting transport to hospital.

Scalds

Scalds have a similar effect on the skin to burns, but are caused by moist heat such as boiling water, steam or hot oil. Scalds caused by steam are often more severe than those caused by boiling water due to the latent heat given out as the steam condenses to water at 100°C.

Eye injuries

Small hairs or dust in the eyes

Locate the foreign body by pulling down the lower eyelid. Remove the object with the corner of a clean handkerchief or a twist of cotton wool soaked in water. If it is thought to be under the upper lid, lift the upper lid over the lower one so that the lower lashes sweep the inner surface of the upper lid, or let the patient blink the eye under water using an eye bath. If unsuccessful, cover the eye with a sterile eye pad and take the patient to hospital.

Chemicals in the eye

In the salon many hairdressing preparations such as perm lotions, shampoos, conditioners and bleaches may cause painful irritation of the eyeball if they accidentally enter the eye. Treat all cases by flushing the eye with large quantities of water poured gently from a jug, taking care that it does not enter the unaffected eye.

Fractures and sprains

A fracture (a broken bone) or a sprain may occasionally occur as a result of a fall in the salon.

Fractures

These result in the loss of use, swelling and often distortion of the affected limb. The patient should not be moved but should be kept warm while awaiting the arrival of an ambulance. Do not give food or drink as the patient may require an anaesthetic for the setting of the bone.

Sprains

These are due to the tearing of ligaments or other tissues found in a joint, such as the ankle or wrist. Apply a crepe bandage and keep it wet with cold water to reduce any swelling. If the sprain is severe take the patient to hospital for an X-ray in case a bone is fractured.

Hysterical attacks

Nervous, highly excitable people are sometimes subject to hysterical attacks in times of emotional stress, but they usually like an audience and the attacks do not occur when the person is alone. The patient may laugh or cry uncontrollably, roll on the floor, or clutch at other people. Speak firmly without bullying and take the patient out of the salon to a quiet room. When sufficient control has been regained, keep the patient occupied.

UNCONSCIOUSNESS

There are many reasons for unconsciousness, including concussion, diabetic coma, electric shock, epilepsy, fainting, heart attacks, poisoning and strokes. It may be difficult for the hairdresser to detect the cause, but the following general treatment should be carried out.

First make sure that the person can breathe freely, that the air passages are not blocked and that there is no restrictive clothing at the neck, waist or chest. Do not leave the patient, but ask someone to telephone for an ambulance immediately. If breathing normally, turn the patient on to one side with the upper arm at right angles to the body and the elbow bent, and the upper leg at right angles to the body with the knee bent.

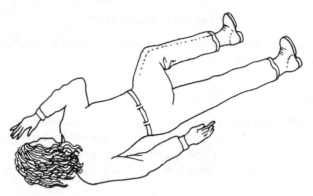

Fig. 4.3   Recovery position

This position prevents the patient from rolling over on to the back and ensures that the air passages stay open and the person is not choked by the tongue or by swallowed saliva or vomit. This three-quarters prone position is known as the **recovery position** and is shown in Fig. 4.3. Observe the patient constantly in case breathing begins to fail and artificial respiration is required. Do not attempt to give food or drink to an unconscious person to avoid choking. Keep the patient warm by covering with a blanket until the ambulance arrives, but do not give a hot-water bottle as this brings blood to the surface of the skin leaving less for vital internal organs.

Artificial respiration

Artificial respiration (mouth-to-mouth resuscitation) must be started at once as soon as breathing begins to fail, because lack of oxygen to the brain for more than a very few minutes would result in permanent brain damage. First ensure that the air passages are open by placing the casualty on her back, pressing the head backwards and the lower jaw upwards as shown in Fig. 4.4. The patient's tongue is thus prevented from falling to the back of the throat so causing blockage of the airway from the mouth and nose to the lungs.

After taking a deep breath surround the patient's mouth completely with your own lips, and at the same time pinch the patient's nostrils together with your fingers. Blow into the patient's lungs, stopping as soon as the chest has risen and then remove your mouth. Repeat the inflation of the lungs at your natural breathing rate until the patient starts breathing again or medical aid is obtained.

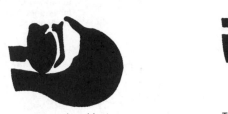
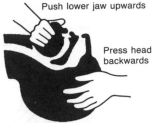

Push lower jaw upwards

Press head backwards

Air passages closed by tongue

To open the air passages

Fig. 4.4 Preparation for mouth to mouth resuscitation

Concussion

This is caused by a blow to the head, possibly by striking the head on furniture when accidentally falling. The patient may be dazed or completely unconscious for a short time and may also suffer shock, so feeling sick and cold. Lay the patient down and cover with a blanket. Carry out the general treatment if the patient is unconscious and obtain medical aid.

Diabetic coma

Diabetes is caused by lack of insulin, a substance secreted by the pancreas which controls the level of sugar in the blood stream. A diabetic coma may result from either a **lack of insulin**, in which case the face would be flushed and the breathing deep with the breath smelling of acetone (nail enamel), or an **excess of insulin** when the skin would be pale and moist, and the breathing shallow but with no smell of acetone.

If still conscious, the patient may recover if given sugar lumps or a strongly sweetened drink. If the patient is unconscious apply the general treatment and send for an ambulance.

Electric shock

Contact with faulty equipment which is not properly earthed can lead to severe injury. The current causes violent contraction of muscle and the person may be unable to break contact with the live apparatus. The severity of the injury depends on the path the current takes as it passes to earth through the body. Breathing may stop due to paralysis of the muscles of respiration, and paralysis of the heart muscles may result in

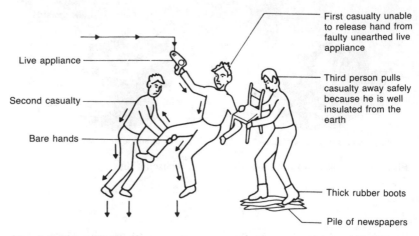

Fig. 4.5 Electric shock

immediate death. Deep burns may also occur, but breathing should always be restored before burns are treated. On no account touch a person in contact with a live apparatus without first insulating yourself (see Fig. 4.5).

If possible switch off the current by removing the plug or by the main switch. The flex may be wrenched from the plug but must never be cut by scissors or a knife. If it is impossible to disconnect the current, insulate yourself with any dry insulating material. Stand on a pile of magazines or wear thick rubber-soled shoes and move the person away from the appliance with dry folded newspapers or a wooden (not metal) chair, protecting the hands with thick rubber gloves if possible.

If breathing has stopped apply artificial respiration, which may need to be continued for some time. If you are alone do not stop to telephone for help until breathing is restored. Send for an ambulance as soon as possible.

Epilepsy

Epilepsy is a recurring condition often first appearing in young people. Fits vary in severity, the mildest involving only momentary loss of consciousness. In more severe cases, the patient may fall unconscious and after a few minutes the limbs may jerk violently due to uncontrollable contractions of the muscles. Do not restrain the movements, but prevent damage to the person by removing surrounding objects such as furniture. Place a knotted handkerchief in the patient's mouth to prevent the biting of the tongue. After the attack keep the patient warm and quiet to encourage sleep.

Fainting

Fainting is a common cause of unconsciousness and is due to an insufficient supply of blood to the brain. It may occur suddenly due to bad news or severe pain, or gradually due to fatigue or to sitting too long in a hot stuffy salon. If the person feels faint, loss of consciousness can often be avoided by lowering the head between the knees or using smelling salts. Increasing the supply of fresh air and unfastening tight clothing will also help. If the patient has fainted, lay the patient down with the head lower than the feet to increase the blood flow to the brain. Unconsciousness is usually brief and a drink of tea or sips of water may be given on recovery.

Heart attacks

Severe pains in the chest, spreading to the arms, neck and the lower part of the face, are the symptoms leading to a heart attack. The patient may be short of breath and suffer serious shock resulting in unconsciousness. If still conscious support the person in a sitting position and loosen any tight clothing at the neck, chest or waist. Immediate hospital treatment is required. If breathing begins to fail commence artificial respiration at once. Test the pulse in the carotid artery in the neck alongside the larynx and if you are certain that there is no pulse and that the heart has therefore stopped beating, alternate breathing into the lungs with pressure over the heart. Place one hand on top of the other over the lower part of the breast bone and press the bone regularly at the rate of one press per second. Alternate one breath into the lungs with five to seven presses over the heart until the ambulance arrives.

Poisoning

A person suspected of having swallowed any type of poison should be conveyed to hospital as quickly as possible and the bottle which held the poison should also be sent along for examination. If a **corrosive** substance such as strong ammonium hydroxide or household bleach has been swallowed, the lips and mouth will show white burns or blisters. In this case give large quantities of water or milk to drink to dilute the poison, and do not attempt to make the patient vomit or further damage to the oesophagus may result. If **non-corrosive** poisons such as overdoses of sleeping tablets or aspirin have been taken and the person is still conscious, try to cause vomiting by tickling the back of the throat with your fingers or a spoon. Do not let this delay dispatch to hospital which may be by car if available. According to current medical opinion, attempts to cause vomiting by drinking an emetic solution of salt and water are dangerous and should not be practised. If unconscious, place the person in the recovery position so that choking is avoided if vomiting occurs. Keep the patient warm by covering with a blanket while waiting for the ambulance. If breathing shows signs of failing apply artificial respiration immediately.

Strokes

Strokes are most common in middle-aged or elderly people and are caused either by bleeding from a burst blood vessel into the brain or by a blood clot blocking a blood vessel to the brain. The symptoms vary from loss of feeling or use of a limb, or slurred speech, to complete unconsciousness. Telephone for an ambulance immediately, and apply the general treatment for unconsciousness if necessary.

FIRST AID BOX

All salons should have a first aid box and an accident register. The minimum contents of the box vary according to the number of employees as laid down in the **Health and Safety (First Aid) Regulations 1981**. The box should be marked with a green cross on a white background and should be closed tightly to keep out dust and moisture. For a salon with fewer than five employees the minimum contents are

- a first aid guidance card
- 10 individually wrapped sterile adhesive dressings
- 1 sterile eye pad
- 1 triangular bandage
- 3 medium unmedicated sterile dressings
- 1 large unmedicated sterile dressing
- 1 extra large unmedicated sterile dressing
- 6 safety pins
- 1 sterile covering for serious wounds.

Useful additions include

- medical wipes

- cotton wool
- a crepe bandage
- tweezers
- disposable gloves for blood spills.

The contents of a first aid box should be replaced as soon as they have been used.

SELF TESTING

1. Why should cuts and abrasions on a hairdresser's hands be kept covered?
2. How would you deal safely with spilled blood?
3. Why is it useful to know a client's medical history?
4. How would you treat a person whose nose was bleeding?
5. What treatment should be given for minor burns and scalds?
6. Give possible reasons for unconsciousness and state how you would treat an unconscious person.
7. What action would you take in a case where breathing had stopped?
8. How would you deal with a person unable to break contact with a live electrical appliance?
9. What treatment should be given to (a) a person who has fainted and (b) a person who was feeling faint?
10. How would you proceed if your client developed severe chest pains?
11. How would you treat a person who had swallowed (a) bleach (b) a large number of aspirins?
12. What action would you take if your client suffered loss of use of a limb and developed slurred speech?

5

ELECTRICAL SAFETY DEVICES

Many salon appliances are powered by electricity and a basic understanding of electrical circuits and electric current helps to ensure safe and efficient handling of appliances. Certain safety features, such as insulation, fuses and earth wires, are included in all salon electrical circuits and a knowledge of their purpose is essential.

WHAT IS ELECTRICITY?

If a nylon brush is used on dry, newly washed hair, the hairs spring apart, tend to cling to the brush and follow its movements. The hair is difficult to manage because it has become charged with electricity. The production of this electrical charge is explained by studying the structure of atoms.

All atoms are made up of two different types of electrically charged particles. Positively charged particles, called **protons**, lie in the nucleus of the atom and negatively charged particles, called **electrons**, move in orbit round the nucleus. Each atom thus resembles a miniature solar system (see Fig. 5.1).

The atoms of each different element have a different number of circulating electrons, but each atom is electrically neutral because the number of negatively charged orbital electrons is balanced by an equal number of positively charged protons in the nucleus. Electrons are much lighter than protons and are more easily removed from the atom.

The friction of rubbing a brush along the hair removes electrons from atoms in the hair. These electrons collect on the brush, giving it a negative charge. Loss of electrons leaves the hair positively charged. Like charges repel each other and opposite charges attract each other, and so the hairs fly apart but are attracted to the brush (see Fig. 5.2). The electrical charges on the brush and hair are known as **static electricity** because

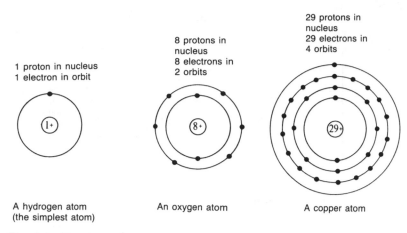

1 proton in nucleus
1 electron in orbit

8 protons in
nucleus
8 electrons in
2 orbits

29 protons in
nucleus
29 electrons in
4 orbits

A hydrogen atom
(the simplest atom)

An oxygen atom

A copper atom

Fig. 5.1   Structure of atoms

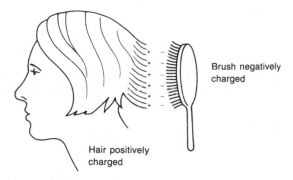

Brush negatively
charged

Hair positively
charged

Fig. 5.2   Static electricity

the electricity is stationary, or sometimes as **frictional electricity** because
the electricity is produced by friction between two substances.

If such electrons can be made to move from atom to atom through
a substance, for example through a copper wire, we call the flow of
electrons an **electric current** (see Fig. 5.3). A flow of electrons through
wires or cables can be produced by a battery or by a power station
generator.

CONDUCTORS AND INSULATORS

Substances through which an electric current will pass easily are said
to be **good conductors** of electricity, e.g. silver and copper. Substances

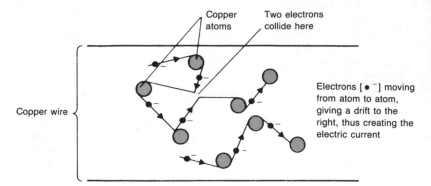

Fig. 5.3   An electric current in a copper wire

which will not allow the passage of an electric current are called **insulators**, e.g. rubber and plastic.

Copper wires are used to carry electricity in electrical cables and in the flexes of electrical appliances. They are surrounded by rubber or plastic insulation to keep the current safely in the wires and prevent it from passing into the human body so causing electric shock. The outer covers of switches, plugs and sockets are usually plastic too. The outside bodywork of some hair dryers is **all-insulated** by being made entirely of plastic.

Safety notes

- Flexes with worn insulation must be replaced. Bare wires can cause electric shock.
- Broken or cracked plugs must be replaced. Cracked sockets and cracked switches must be replaced by an electrician.
- Water can bypass insulation and carry an electric current. Never touch electrical equipment with wet hands.

ELECTRICAL CIRCUITS

An electric current will flow only if there is a complete conducting path from the source of electricity (a battery or the generator at a power station) through an appliance and back again to the source. This pathway is called a circuit. A switch is used to complete the circuit (switch on) or break the circuit (switch off). The circuit in Fig. 5.4 is powered by a battery

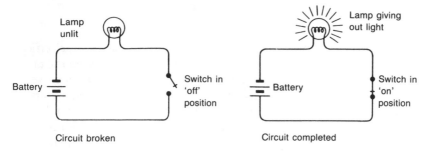

Fig. 5.4 Electrical circuits

and shows how a bulb can be switched on and off or how the circuit can be completed and broken. Salon circuits work in a similar way, though the electricity comes from a power station instead of a battery.

MAINS ELECTRICITY

Mains electricity, generated at a power station, is carried along overhead cables held by pylons and finally enters buildings by underground cables. The current may be regarded as travelling from the power station to a salon along a feed cable or live wire and returning to the power station by a return or neutral wire. The circuit is completed when an appliance is plugged in and switched on (see Fig. 5.5). Switches are always installed in the live wire.

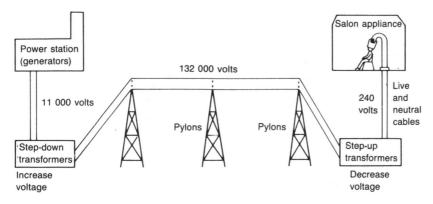

Fig. 5.5 Mains electricity supply

VOLTAGE

Both batteries and mains generators act like pumps which force electricity through the wiring and can be compared with the way a mechanical pump forces water through water pipes (see Fig. 5.6). The **electrical pressure** produced is called the **voltage** and is measured in units called **volts**. A small torch battery would produce 1.5 volts sufficient for a torch bulb but not sufficient to operate a hair dryer. The huge voltage produced by a mains generator (11 000 volts) is reduced to 240 volts before reaching a salon (see Fig. 5.5) and this is the voltage at which salon appliances work.

It is important to use appliances at the correct voltage. Some foreign appliances are designed to be used at 110 volts (the normal voltage in some other countries) and would be damaged if plugged into a 240 voltage supply. If you buy foreign appliances make sure they are designed for a 240 volt supply. Electric shavers are sometimes designed to work at

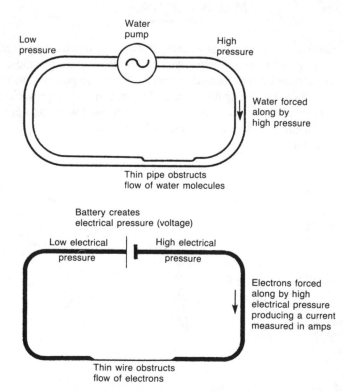

Fig. 5.6 Comparison between voltage and water pressure

either 110 or 240 volts by use of a switch. The voltage at which an appliance should be used is normally indicated on the appliance.

SALON CIRCUITS

In a salon, underground cables lead electricity first to the Electricity Board's sealed fuse box. This box must only be opened by the Board's engineers. Next to the sealed box is the **meter** (recording how much current is used) and the **consumer unit** which contains the main switch and main fuses or circuit breakers (which are a more modern alternative to fuses). Several individual circuits radiate from the fuses or the circuit breakers, including the lighting circuit, one or more circuits for power plugs and often separate circuits for immersion heaters or instantaneous water heaters (see Fig. 5.7). Electric storage heaters and water heaters may be time controlled to operate only during cheap night-rate periods: these are connected to a separate consumer unit and fitted with a time switch. Power circuits are in the form of a closed loop called a **ring main circuit** which goes from room to room round the salon. Sockets may be wired into the ring main at any desired point by an electrician.

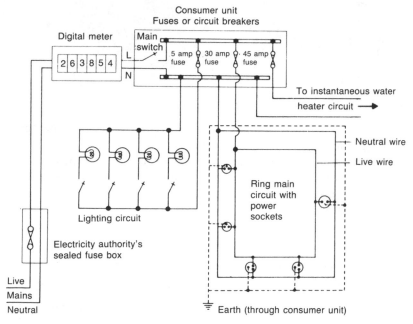

Fig. 5.7 Salon circuit

Safety note

- It is important to know the position of the main switch for the salon. In an emergency, such as accident, fire or flood, it can be used to switch off the whole of the salon supply. It should be switched off when replacing circuit fuses in the main fuse box.

Wiring

The electrical cables for salon circuits lie mainly behind the plaster of the walls or under the floorboards, though in modern installations they may be fitted in plastic channels or trunking laid over the plaster at skirting level so allowing easy access for later modifications. The only visible parts of the circuits are socket outlets and switches. Insulated copper wiring is used for circuit cables, but the thickness of the wire varies according to the size of current the particular cable is designed to carry. The size of a current is measured in units called **amperes** (A or amps). The thick cable used in a circuit for an instantaneous water heater may be designed to carry a current up to 45 amps, a ring main circuit 30 amps, but a lighting circuit only 5 amps. If a cable carries a greater current than that for which it was designed it is said to be **overloaded**.

OVERLOADING

Overloading can be caused in three main ways:

- Plugging too many appliances into a circuit by using an adaptor to plug several appliances into one socket.
- Using too many appliances at the same time in a ring main circuit. The numerous sockets in a ring main are for convenience and to avoid long trailing flexes, and it is assumed that not all the sockets will be in use at any one time.
- Connecting heating or power appliances into a lighting circuit.

Overloading may cause the wiring to get hot and may start a fire, possibly under the floorboards. The circuit fuse is designed as a safety device to prevent this from happening by cutting off the current if overloading takes place.

CIRCUIT FUSES

The consumer unit contains a fuse for each circuit (see Fig. 5.7). The fuse is a safety device consisting of a short length of wire which is designed to be the weakest part of the circuit. The fuse wire will get hot and melt if the current in the circuit exceeds the safety limit for that circuit. The melting of the fuse creates a break in the circuit and so cuts off the current. This protects the wiring from overheating and prevents a possible outbreak of fire. The fuse always forms part of the live wire of the circuit. Each circuit fuse has a rating (in amps) depending on the maximum size of current the circuit is required to carry. A lighting circuit contains a very fine fuse wire with a current rating of 5 amps, so that the fuse would melt if the current exceeded 5 amps. A ring main circuit for power appliances has a thicker fuse wire with a current rating of 30 amps and an instantaneous water heater circuit one of 45 amps.

Blown fuses

The circuit fuse may melt or 'blow' due to three main causes:

- Overloading the circuit.
- Faulty wiring: worn insulation may lead to a **short circuit** if the live wire touches either the neutral or the earth wire, as the appliance is bypassed, causing a large surge of current. A short circuit may also occur if cables are pierced when driving nails into plaster or into floorboards.
- Old or corroded fuse wire.

A blown fuse must be replaced but only after the fault has been located and corrected, or the fuse will blow again. To repair a circuit fuse, disconnect all appliances, switch off the main switch, open the consumer unit and locate the blown fuse by removing the appropriate holder. There are two kinds: rewirable fuses and cartridge fuses.

Rewirable fuses

In rewirable fuses, the fuse wire is threaded through a ceramic carrier or tube and secured by two screws. The carrier or tube is held in a plastic holder. To repair this type of fuse, discard any old fuse wire held in the screws and rethread new fuse wire of the correct size for the circuit, through the ceramic holder. Secure the wire under the screws, being careful not to stretch the wire when tightening the second screw. Cut off any spare wire. Replace the fuse holder and switch on the main switch. Time will be saved if a card of fuse wire containing several sizes of fuse wire is kept in readiness near the consumer unit.

Cartridge fuses

Cartridge fuses consist of a fuse wire contained in a small ceramic tube and attached to metal caps at each end of the fuse (see Fig. 5.8). The tube contains sand in case sparking occurs when the fuse blows. The cartridge fits into spring clips in the fuse holder. The current rating is stamped on the side of the fuse. This type is more modern than rewirable fuses and is easier to replace by inserting a new cartridge of the correct value into the spring clips.

Safety note

- It is important to use the correct size of fuse wire or cartridge. If the current rating of the fuse is too high the cables will overheat before the fuse melts and may cause fire.

CIRCUIT BREAKERS

In modern electrical installations the consumer unit contains circuit breakers instead of fuses (see Fig. 5.9). The circuit breaker is an automatic switch which cuts off the supply whenever excess current flows through the circuit, due either to a fault or overloading. The current can be restored simply by switching to the 'on' position when the overload has been cleared or the faulty appliance removed. This is much quicker than replacing a fuse and the installation of circuit breakers is very advantageous in a busy salon.

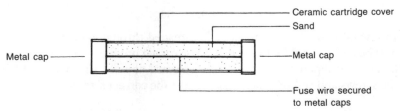

Fig. 5.8 Cartridge fuse

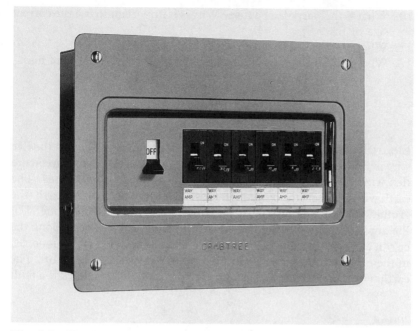

Fig. 5.9   Circuit breakers

The consumer unit may also be fitted with a residual current device or current operated earth-leakage circuit breaker which immediately cuts off the power supply on detecting any leakage of current to earth. It is thus a safeguard against electric shock and fire due to electrical faults.

SELF TESTING

1. What is meant by static electricity?
2. Name the negatively charged particles which form the flow of an electric current.
3. What is meant by an insulator? Give two examples of substances which are good insulators.
4. Why should flexes with worn insulation be replaced?
5. Why is it dangerous to use electrical equipment with wet hands?
6. What is meant by an electrical circuit?
7. What is the size of mains voltage in the United Kingdom?
8. What is meant by overloading a circuit and what is the likely effect of overloading?
9. What is meant by a short circuit? How may a short circuit be caused?

10. What is the purpose of a fuse? Why is it important to use the correct size of fuse?
11. What are the causes of a blown fuse?
12. What is the advantage of installing circuit breakers instead of fuses?

THE EARTH WIRE

Electricity may be regarded as being brought to an appliance by the live wire and leaving by the neutral wire. Many appliances have a three-core flex with an **earth wire** in addition to the live and neutral wires. The earth wire connects the outer metal case of an appliance to the earth (the ground). The earth wire must be continuous from the outer metal of the appliance, through the flex, through the plug and socket, along the circuit cable and into the ground under the building, where it is connected to the metal sheath of the Electricity Board's cable (see Fig. 5.10). The earth wire is a safety device designed to prevent electric shock if a fault

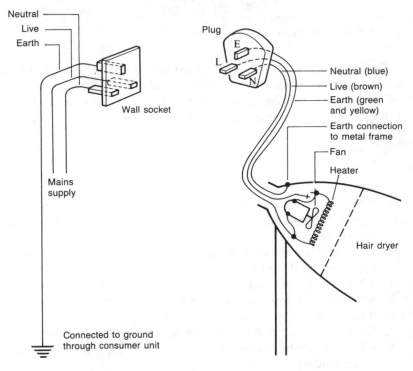

Fig. 5.10   Connection of the earth wire

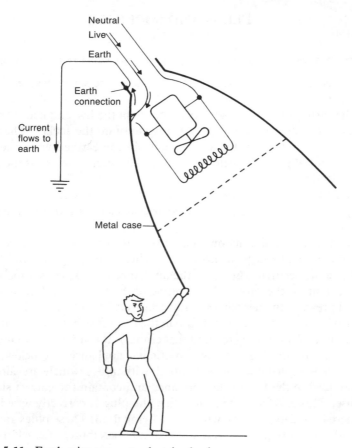

Fig. 5.11   Earth wire prevents electric shock

develops in the appliance. In normal working there is no current flowing through the earth wire.

Due to a loose live wire or to faulty insulation inside an appliance, the outer metal casing of the appliance could become live (see Fig. 5.11). In a correctly earthed appliance the earth wire provides an easier path for the electricity than the passage through the human body and so carries the current safely to earth. In this way a person touching the metal casing would be saved from a possibly fatal electric shock. The passage of the current to earth would also result in a large surge of current causing the fuse to melt so cutting off the current.

All appliances with metal on the outside should be earthed unless they bear the sign ▢ indicating that they are double insulated. In this case any metal is completely insulated on the inside of the appliance and there is no danger of a fault causing the outer casing to become live.

PLUGS AND SOCKETS

There are various safety features in plugs and sockets to ensure safe usage.

- Sockets may be shuttered so that the holes are safely covered when not in use.
- The earth pin, which is always longer than the live and neutral pins, opens the shutters as the plug is inserted into the socket. The long pin also ensures that the appliance is already earthed when the live and neutral pins complete the circuit. The shutters close as the plug is withdrawn.
- In modern plugs the live and neutral pins are insulated except at their tips, to lessen the possibility of electric shock caused by touching the pins when inserting or removing the plug.
- Each plug contains its own cartridge fuse designed to protect the appliance and flex to which it is attached. The plug fuse will blow if a fault, occurring in either the appliance or flex, causes too large a current for the wiring. The melting of the fuse cuts off the current and prevents further damage or overheating. No other appliance will then be affected. (If a circuit fuse in the main fuse box blows it affects all the appliances plugged into that circuit). It is important to use the correct size of plug fuse for a particular appliance (see below).
- All new appliances are now fitted with plugs which are already moulded to the flex of the appliance and contain the correct size of fuse. This is safer as it ensures that the plug is correctly wired and there is no danger of the wrong fuse being used. These plugs are also made of shatterproof plastic to avoid any possibility of cracking the plug cover by misuse.

Safety notes

- Avoid the use of adaptors. Sockets are only designed to carry a current of up to 13 amps and overloading may occur if an adaptor is used to plug several appliances into one socket.
- Take care not to damage plugs by dropping them on to hard surfaces. Plugs with damaged or bent pins may not fit the socket perfectly and may become hot if a spark jumps across any small air gap between plug and socket. Such a plug should be replaced as there is danger of fire.
- Any appliance, plug, socket or flex which is overheating is faulty and requires attention.

Using the correct size of plug fuse

A plug fuse is designed to melt if the current (measured in amps) exceeds the safety limit for the wiring. Plug cartridge fuses are available in current rating of 3 amps, 5 amps, and 13 amps. To decide which size of fuse is required, we need to know the **power of the appliance** to which the plug is attached. The power is the rate at which the appliance uses electricity and is measured in units called **watts**. A high powered light bulb of 250 watts gives a very bright light; a low powered bulb of 15 watts gives a dim light suitable only for decorative purposes. The higher the wattage of the appliance the greater the consumption of electricity in a given time. The power of an appliance is usually marked on a small plate on the appliance along with the voltage at which it is to be used.

Typical wattages for salon appliances:

- hair clippers 20 watts
- steamer 750 watts
- hand hair dryer 500−1000 watts
- hood dryer 1000−2000 watts
- immersion heater 3000 watts
- washing machine with heater 3000 watts

- a 3 amp fuse is used for appliances up to 720 watts
- a 5 amp fuse is used for appliances of 720−1200 watts
- a 13 amp fuse is used for appliances of 1200−3000 watts.

The power of an appliance depends on both the voltage at which it works and the size of the current flowing. The relationship between these quantities can be expressed in two ways:

$$\text{Power} = \text{voltage} \times \text{size of current}$$
$$\text{Watts} = \text{volts} \times \text{amps}$$

To calculate the correct fuse size we need to know the size of the current flowing (amps) when the appliance is plugged into a 240 volt supply.

If watts = volts × amps
the size of current (amps) = watts ÷ volts
The size of the fuse must be greater than the normal current and have a current rating of 3 amps, 5 amps or 13 amps.

Example: Calculate the correct fuse size of plug fuse for a 1000 watt hairdryer on a 240 volt supply.

Size of current through fuse = Watts ÷ volts = 1000 ÷ 240 = 4.2 amps

A 3 amp fuse would be too small for this hairdryer, a 5 amp fuse is required.

Safety note

* When a new plug is bought it may contain a standard 13 amp fuse. This must be replaced if the wattage of the appliance to which it is to be attached is less than 1200 watts. If the fuse rating is too high it will not protect the wiring and this may get hot before the fuse melts. It is essential to use the correct fuse size.

Wiring a plug correctly

The three cores of a flex—live, neutral and earth wires—are coated with different coloured plastic insulation so that it is easy to connect the correct wire to the corresponding terminal in the plug.

The internationally used colour code for the cores is as follows:

* **Brown** to be connected to the terminal marked **live** or **L**
* **Blue** to be connected to the terminal marked **neutral** or **N**
* **Green and yellow** to be connected to the terminal marked **earth** or **E**.

Proceed as follows:

* Cut back the outer insulation to expose the three coloured cores, taking care not to cut the coloured insulation (see Fig. 5.12).
* Strip the core insulation, exposing sufficient bare wire to make a connection so that the insulation just reaches the terminals (see Fig. 5.13).

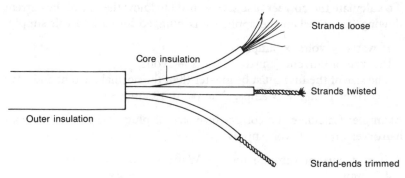

Fig. 5.12   Three-core flex

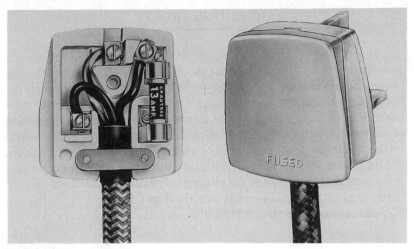

Fig. 5.13 Fused plug

- Twist the strands of wire for each core separately and trim the ends (see Fig. 5.12).
- Screw the cable in place under the cable grip.
- Connect the three cores to the corresponding terminals according to the colour code. If the wire passes round a screw it should do so in a clockwise direction so that the wire stays close to the screw-thread. The insulation should just reach the screw in each case and the screws should be tight.
- Replace the cartridge fuse checking that it is the correct size for the appliance.
- Screw down the plug top.

Safety notes

- Wrong connections in the plug are dangerous. If live and earth wires are interchanged, the metal frame of an appliance would be live. If live and neutral are interchanged, the switch of the appliance would be in the neutral wire and the equipment would remain live even if switched off.
- Use the correct size of fuse.
- Never remove a plug from a socket by pulling the flex. The connections inside the plug may be loosened.
- Avoid long trailing flexes over which people may trip.
- Avoid placing flexes under carpets as insulation may become worn.

ELECTRIC SHOCK

If a person's body completes a mains circuit, the person will experience an electric shock. The effect of the shock will vary according to the size of the current flowing and on the pathway of the current through the body. A small current may produce a tingling feeling, while stronger currents may cause contraction of the muscles and burns. Contraction of the muscles in the arms often prevents the release of the person's grip on the appliance. If the current causes contraction of the heart muscles, the heart may stop beating. Breathing will stop if the diaphragm and intercostal muscles between the ribs are contracted. Immediate first aid is required in both cases and is described in Chapter 4.

A person may complete a circuit in several different ways:

By touching both live and neutral wires

For this situation, see Fig. 5.14.

By touching a live wire and an earthed metal

The earth behaves as an electrical conductor. Metal water pipes which enter the ground provide a path to earth. A person in contact with a live wire and a tap or water pipe may complete a circuit and receive a

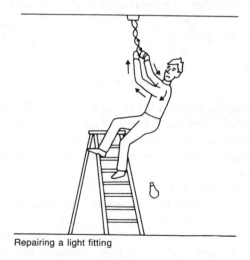

Repairing a light fitting

Fig. 5.14 Effect of touching both live and neutral wires

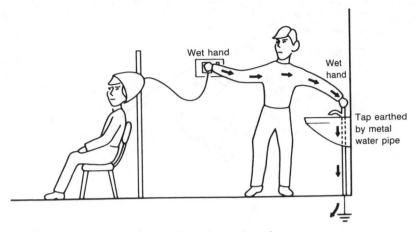

Wet hand

Wet hand

Tap earthed
by metal
water pipe

Fig. 5.15 Effect of touching a live wire and earth

shock. Touching a plug with wet hands has the same effect as touching
a live wire since impure water is a good conductor. If an earthed metal
is touched at the same time, a shock will result (see Fig. 5.15).

By touching a live unearthed metal (or a bare live wire) and the earth

If the outer metal case of an appliance becomes live due to a fault and
the metal is not earthed, a person can complete the circuit through the
ground (see Fig. 5.16). Similarly on touching a bare live wire a person
would receive an electric shock by conducting the current to earth.

SELF TESTING

1. What is the purpose of an earth wire? To what part of an appliance
   would the earth wire be connected?
2. What sign on an appliance would show that no earth wire was
   required?
3. Why is the earth pin of a 3-pin plug longer than the live or neutral
   pins?
4. What is the purpose of a plug fuse? What may cause this fuse to
   blow?
5. Why is it bad practice to plug several appliances into one socket using
   an adaptor?

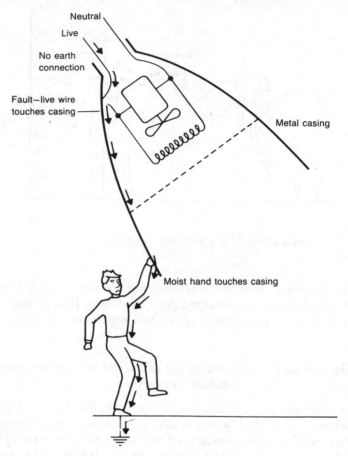

Fig. 5.16 Touching a live unearthed metal

6. What is the international colour coding used when wiring plugs?
7. The figures 240 volts and 450 watts are given on a blow dryer. What do these figures mean? What is the correct size of fuse for the plug of this appliance?
8. What effect can electric shock have on the human body?
9. Mention three ways in which a person may suffer electric shock.
10. Why should you not use electrical equipment while standing on a wet floor?

PART 2
HAIR AND HAIR GROWTH

6

HAIR

Hairdressing is concerned with the care and dressing of the scalp hair. This strong coarse hair is known as **terminal hair** but among it there is always a smaller amount of soft fine hair or **vellus hair**. Fine downy vellus hair also grows from most parts of the skin except the soles of the feet, palms of the hands and the lips. The hair of the human foetus is even finer, and is known as **lanugo hair**, but this is shed about one month before birth when vellus hair starts to grow. Terminal hair usually replaces the vellus hair of the scalp soon after birth, though many babies are born with a considerable amount of terminal scalp hair. At puberty, terminal hair also replaces vellus hair in the armpits (axillae) and in the pubic area. In males, coarse terminal hair grows at this time in the beard and chest areas as well. If the man later becomes bald, vellus hair is again produced on the scalp in place of terminal hair. Short bristle type hairs grow in the nostrils and also form the eyelashes and eyebrows.

WHAT IS HAIR?

The part of the hair that is seen above the surface of the skin is the **hair shaft** and, unless the hair has been cut, the tip is always pointed. The hair shaft is composed of a dead, tough horny protein material called **keratin**. The actively growing and therefore living part of the hair is situated below the surface of the skin at the base of a minute pit (about 4 mm deep and 0.4 mm wide) known as a **hair follicle** (see Fig. 6.1). Thus the hair dies as it grows up the follicle, becomes hardened, and emerges from the surface of the skin as a dead material in the form of keratin. This process of hardening to form keratin is called **keratinization**.

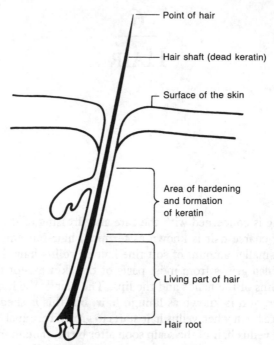

Fig. 6.1 Section of a hair follicle

The labels on the figure are:
- Point of hair
- Hair shaft (dead keratin)
- Surface of the skin
- Area of hardening and formation of keratin
- Living part of hair
- Hair root

LAYERS OF A HAIR

A scalp hair consists of three layers, as shown in Fig. 6.2. This shows a hair cut across its width and one cut along its length. The three layers, from the outside to the centre of the hair, are the cuticle, the cortex and the medulla.

The cuticle

If you take a single hair from your scalp and run your fingers along its length, first in one direction and then in the other, you should notice that it feels slightly rougher when your fingers run towards the end pulled from the scalp (the root end). This is because the outer layer of a hair, the cuticle, consists of **overlapping scales** or imbrications of hard keratin, the tips of which project towards the free end or point of the hair (see Figs. 6.3a and 6.3b). The scales are colourless and translucent (like frosted glass) so that hair colour, due to pigment granules of melanin in the cortex, can be seen through the scales.

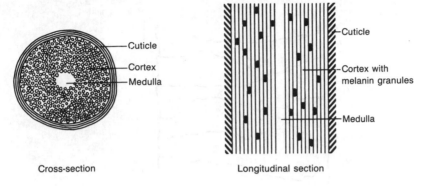

Cross-section   Longitudinal section

Fig. 6.2 Sections of a hair

The scales fit tightly over each other like the tiles on a roof and tend to prevent water and other liquids from entering the hair shaft. They may extend part way round the hair shaft or completely round to form a ring. The edges of the scales are smooth on the newly grown hair near the scalp, but become rougher towards the points where the hair is older. The thickness of the cuticle depends on the degree of overlapping of the scales. This varies from seven to eleven layers (see Fig. 6.4). The structure of the cuticle allows the scales to slip over each other when the hair is stretched as in setting the hair round rollers. This tough outer cuticle serves to hold the whole hair together. The cuticle may be damaged by chemicals or harsh treatment.

The cortex

Immediately under the cuticle is the cortex which forms the main bulk of the hair. The cortex consists of the remains of elongated spindle-shaped cells containing a tough fibrous type of keratin with long bundles or cables of fibres running parallel to the length of the hair. The cells are closely bound together by a cementing material or **matrix**, but there are some air spaces between them. The cortex contains granules of a **pigment** called **melanin** which is mainly responsible for the colour of hair.

The medulla

The central core of the hair, the medulla, consists of a honeycomb of irregularly shaped areas of keratin with many air spaces between them. The medulla is not present in all hairs, particularly if the hair is fine. Sometimes it is not continuous along the whole length of a hair.

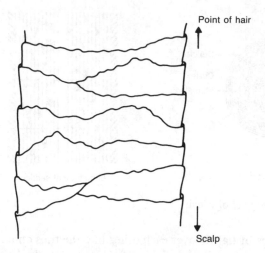

Point of hair

Scalp

Fig. 6.3a   Surface scales of a hair

STRUCTURE OF THE CORTEX

The cortex is the most important part of the hair for it is this layer which is most affected during various hairdressing processes. During bleaching, the coloured melanin in the cortex is changed chemically into a colourless substance by the action of hydrogen peroxide. Permanent dyes penetrate into the cortex to add colour to the hair and the chemical structure of the cortex is changed during permanent waving.

By the use of the scanning electron microscope and by X-ray methods, scientists have been able to study the structure of the keratin of the cortex (see Fig. 6.5a). It consists of a series of fibres containing even finer fibres. The largest fibres, or **macrofibrils**, lying parallel to the length of the hair, are held together by a matrix of twisted keratin fibres and by the interlocking of protruding fibrils (see Fig. 6.5b).

The macrofibrils are made up of smaller fibres called **microfibrils** which in turn contain **protofibrils**. Each protofibril consists of a group of three coiled chains known as **polypeptide chains**. The chains have a spiral shape called an **alpha-helix** (alpha, written α, is the first letter of the Greek alphabet) and are like minute coiled springs held together by cross linkages in a ladder-like structure (see Fig. 6.6).

Boiling hair with hydrochloric acid splits the polypeptide chains into chemical substances called **amino acids** of which there are eighteen different types in keratin. Each amino acid consists of a different arrangement of the **chemical elements** carbon, hydrogen, oxygen and nitrogen chemically united together. Two of the amino acids, cystine and cysteine, also contain the element sulphur in addition to the other

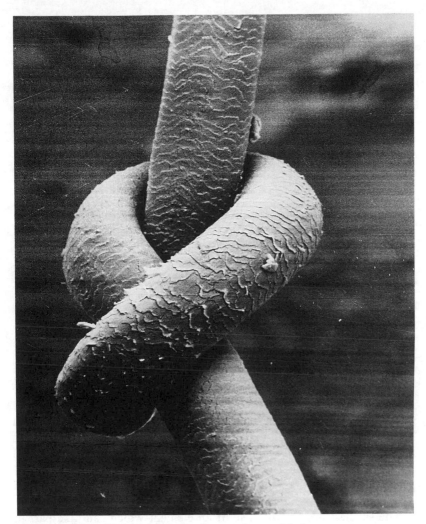

Fig. 6.3b Magnified photograph of an undamaged hair

four elements mentioned. This is important in the study of perming.
The elements in keratin are present in the following proportion:

Carbon 50 per cent
Oxygen 21 per cent
Nitrogen 18 per cent
Hydrogen 7 per cent
Sulphur 4 per cent

In common with all chemical elements, these substances cannot be split
into any simpler substances.

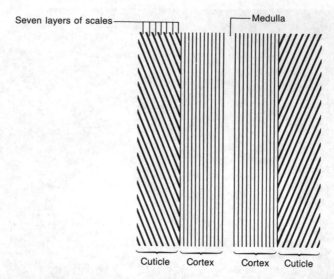

Fig. 6.4   Section of hair showing overlapping cuticle scales

ELEMENTS AND COMPOUNDS

A knowledge of the meaning of elements, compounds, atoms and molecules is necessary in order to fully understand the chemical structure of keratin.

The five elements of hair keratin are among a total of about a hundred different elements which exist. **Elements** are the simplest susbtances obtainable and may be regarded as the building bricks from which all things, including living organisms, are made. They join together by chemical reaction to form more complicated substances called **compounds**.

The smallest possible particle of an element which can take part in a chemical reaction is an **atom** of that element. The atoms of any one element are all alike but are different from the atoms of all other elements. A **molecule** consists of two or more atoms chemically united together and is the smallest part of a substance which can exist by itself.

Water and hydrogen peroxide are two quite simple compounds and both contain the same two elements, oxygen and hydrogen. Each molecule of water contains two atoms of hydrogen combined with one atom of oxygen. The chemical formula of water is written H_2O. Each molecule of hydrogen peroxide contains two atoms of hydrogen combined with two atoms of oxygen. The chemical formula of hydrogen peroxide is written H_2O_2. Hydrogen peroxide is used in many hairdressing

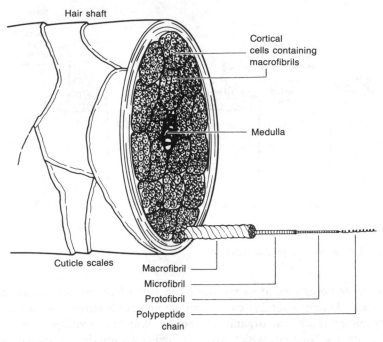

Fig. 6.5a Structure of the cortex

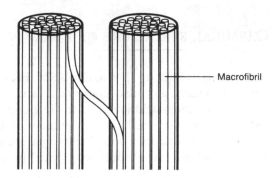

Fig. 6.5b Interlocking protruding fibrils

processes including bleaching, permanent colouring, and neutralizing after perming. During these chemical processes each molecule of hydrogen peroxide gives one of its oxygen atoms to another substance, leaving a molecule of water. A substance like hydrogen peroxide, which can give oxygen to another substance during a chemical reaction, is called an **oxidizing agent**.

Hair keratin is a much more complicated compound than water or

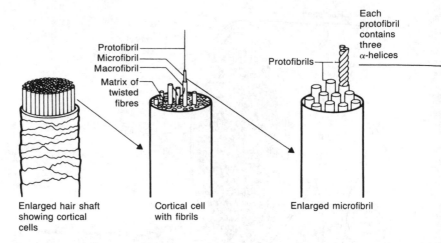

Fig. 6.6 Structure of hair keratin

hydrogen peroxide and its molecule contains a large number of atoms. Because keratin contains carbon atoms and is obtained from a living organism it is called an **organic compound**. Water and hydrogen peroxide and other substances which are obtained from non-living sources are called **inorganic compounds**.

CHEMICAL STRUCTURE OF KERATIN

Keratin, like all proteins, is built up from **amino acids**. Each amino acid molecule consists of two parts: an amino group and an acid group. When the amino group of one amino acid joins the acidic group of another, a **peptide bond** or linkage is formed. A large number of amino acids joined together in this way by peptide bonds forms a **polypeptide chain**.

The formation of a polypeptide chain is represented in the diagram.

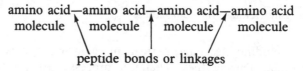

Each protofibril in the cortex consists of a group of three such polypeptide chains (see Fig. 6.6). The chains have a spiral or coiled spring shape known as an **α-helix** with three or four amino acids in each turn of the coil. The three polypeptide chains are connected by several different types of cross linkages or bonds to form a ladder-like structure (see Fig. 6.7).

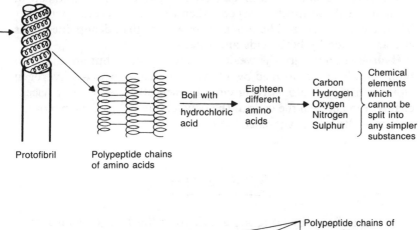

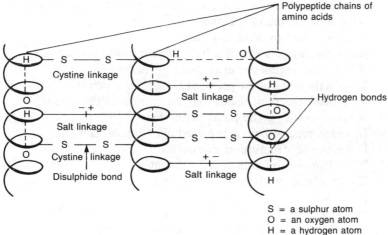

Fig. 6.7   Polypeptide chains with cross linkages

The bonds in keratin are important in perming and setting hair. They may be damaged by overprocessing during bleaching and perming, leading to loss of condition of the hair and possibly to breakage of the hair itself.

Cystine linkages are the strongest of the cross linkages in keratin. Each molecule of the amino acid cystine forms part of two adjacent polypeptide chains with the cystine linkage making a bridge between the chains. The cystine linkages each contain two sulphur atoms which are held by a **disulphide bond**. This type of bond takes part in chemical reactions during perming.

Salt linkages or bonds are due to electrostatic attraction between the acid part of one amino acid (negatively charged) and the amino part of an amino acid (positively charged) when these lie opposite each other in the adjacent chains. These bonds are weaker than disulphide bonds and are broken by both acids and alkalis.

Hydrogen bonds are the weakest of all the bonds but are the most numerous. They are formed by a force of attraction between hydrogen atoms and oxygen atoms lying close to each other, either in adjacent chains or in between the coils of the polypeptide chains. The bonds are broken if the hair is stretched.

SELF TESTING

1. What is meant by (a) terminal hair (b) vellus hair (c) lanugo hair?
2. What is the name of the protein of hair?
3. What is meant by keratinization?
4. Name the three layers of a hair, starting from the outside.
5. Which layer forms the main bulk of the hair?
6. What is the name of the pigment of hair? In which layer is it found?
7. How many layers of scales may be present in the cuticle?
8. What is meant by the point of the hair?
9. In which type of hair is the medulla often missing?
10. Describe the structure of the cortex.
11. What is meant by a chemical element?
12. Which chemical elements are present in (a) hair (b) hydrogen peroxide?
13. How many different types of amino acids are present in hair keratin?
14. Name two amino acids which contain the element sulphur.
15. What is meant by an organic compound?
16. Name three types of bonds or cross-linkages in keratin. Which bond is (a) strongest (b) weakest?
17. What shape is a polypeptide chain? Of what does the chain consist?
18. Name the type of bond present in a polypeptide chain.

PHYSICAL PROPERTIES OF HAIR

The physical properties of a substance include its appearance, feel, and behaviour which does not involve a chemical reaction.

Colour of hair

Hair colour depends on the number and kind of pigment granules in the cortex. The cuticle is translucent so that the colour shows through. Black and brown hairs contain the pigment **melanin**; blonde hairs contain the yellow-red pigment **pheomelanin**; white hairs have little or no pigment; grey hair is considered to be a mixture of white and coloured hairs. Most hairs contain a mixture of pigments.

Elasticity of hair

The elasticity of hair is due to the coiled spring structure of keratin. Hair will stretch and then spring back when released. Elasticity increases if the hair is wet. If it is over-stretched it reaches its **elastic limit** and loses the ability to spring back. If stretched beyond this limit, the hair may break. The force required to break the hair is a measure of its **tensile strength**. Wet hair has greater elasticity than dry hair but its tensile strength is lower, so a dry hair will support a greater weight before breaking.

The elasticity of hair can be shown by preparing a bundle of about ten hairs each approximately 20 cm long and knotting the hairs together at each end. After soaking the bundle in water containing a little shampoo, hold one end in each hand. On pulling firmly, the hairs may be felt and seen to stretch and to spring back when released.

Elasticity is important when setting hair and will be considered more fully in Chapter 13 on Setting and Drying. A satisfactory set cannot be achieved unless elasticity is good.

Porosity of hair

Liquids may pass between the cuticle scales into the cortex, the porosity depending on the state of the cuticle. If the cuticle has been damaged or if the scales have been lifted by treatment with dry heat, steam or alkalis, the porosity is increased. Substances coating the hair shaft, such as the natural oils of the scalp, conditioning creams or lacquer, decrease the porosity. Hair is more porous towards its points due to normal wear and tear through brushing and combing, and also to possible chemical damage if the hair has been permed, bleached or tinted.

Porosity is important in perming and colouring because porous hair may soak up chemicals too quickly. Chemicals are drawn up by **capillary action** into the narrow air spaces of the cortex. Pre-treatment is sometimes

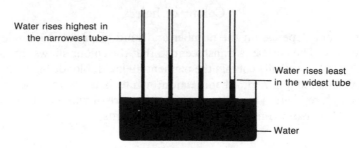

Fig. 6.8 Capillary rise

necessary to even out the porosity of the hair and will be considered again in Chapters 14 and 15 on Permanent Waving and Colouring Hair.

Capillary rise can be illustrated by supporting several glass capillary tubes of different bore in a dish of coloured water as shown in Fig. 6.8. The water rises highest in the narrowest tube. This effect is due to a force of attraction between the water molecules and the molecules of the glass. Liquids rise in the narrow spaces of the cortex in a similar way.

Thickness of hair

A hair is usually the same thickness or diameter all along its length. An average diameter is 0.05 millimetres. If soaked in water, a hair increases in thickness by a greater proportion than it increases in length. This is due to water being drawn into the air spaces between the fibres of the cortex by capillary action and causing the hair to swell.

A microscope can be used to compare the thickness and colour of hairs by placing several hairs from different heads on to a microscope slide and adding a drop of water or glycerine to help hold the hairs in place. After covering with a cover-slip the slide is examined under a microscope and differences in colour and thickness of the hairs noted. Repeat using several hairs from the same head. Cut a single hair into two pieces and soak one in water for several hours. Mount both pieces on the same slide and examine for variation in thickness. The actual thickness of hair can be measured with the aid of a microscope scale.

Hair is hygroscopic

Since hair absorbs moisture easily from the air it is said to be hygroscopic. The normal moisture content of hair is 10 per cent by weight, but it may be as high as 30 per cent. The presence of moisture in the hair makes it more pliable and elastic. Gradual absorption of moisture from the air will destroy a set. Absorption can be reduced by the use of setting lotions and lacquer.

Hair can be shown to be hygroscopic by weighing a quantity of hair clippings in an evaporating dish and placing the dish in an oven at 110°C for several hours. Reweigh the dish after cooling in a desiccator and note the loss of weight. Next leave the dish to stand overnight in the air. Reweigh and note the gain in weight.

Texture of hair

A combination of some of the properties already mentioned determines the texture or feel of hair which depends on

- the thickness of the hair
- the degree of roughness of the cuticle
- the moisture level of the cortex
- the length of the hair: very short hair seems stiff, while long hair seems softer.

CHEMICAL PROPERTIES OF HAIR

Action of acids and alkalis on hair

Hair reacts differently to the two groups of chemical substances known as **acids** and **alkalis,** and their identification in hairdressing preparations is therefore important. The presence of acids and alkalis may be detected by the change in colour of an **indicator paper** impregnated with **litmus** dye. Red litmus paper turns blue in alkaline liquids and blue litmus paper turns red in acids. The use of **universal** indicator paper (**pH** paper) not only shows the presence of acids or alkalis, but also indicates the strength of the acid or alkali by changing through a wide range of colours corresponding to a numerical pH scale of 0 to 14 (see Fig. 6.9). Values below 7 indicate acidity (the lower the number the stronger the acid), while values of 7 to 14 indicate increasing alkalinity. A substance which is neither acid nor alkaline is **neutral** and has a pH of 7.

The term pH means the power of hydrogen ions. In water, molecules of acids and alkalis split to form electrically charged particles called **ions.** Acids always produce positively charged hydrogen ions (H^+). The greater the number of hydrogen ions the stronger the acid and the lower the pH value.

Alkalis produce negatively charged hydroxyl ions (OH^-). The greater the concentration of hydroxyl ions, the more alkaline the solution and

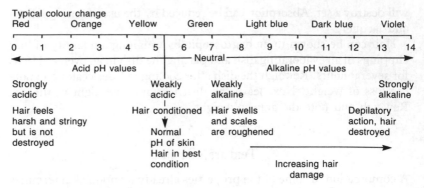

Fig. 6.9 The pH scale

the higher the pH value. If an alkali is added to an acid, the hydroxyl ions will tend to combine with the hydrogen ions to produce water so reducing acidity.

$$H^+ \quad + \quad OH^- \quad \longrightarrow \quad H_2O$$

hydrogen   hydroxyl   water
ion   ion   molecule

When the number of hydroxyl ions and the number of hydrogen ions is equal the solution is neutral with a pH of 7.

Inorganic acids

Inorganic or mineral acids, such as sulphuric acid, hydrochloric acid and phosphoric acid, are strong acids used in the laboratory and in the manufacture of other chemical compounds such as soapless detergents. Strong acids with a pH of 1–2 will burn the skin and damage cotton fabrics. They make hair feel harsh and stringy, but do not destroy it unless the hair is boiled with the acid. They are not used by themselves in the salon or on hair.

Organic acids

Organic acids such as citric acid (found in lemon juice), acetic acid (in vinegar), tartaric acid (in grapes) and lactic acid (in milk) are weak acids and dilute solutions may be used directly on the hair. Weak acids with a pH of 5–6 have a conditioning effect on hair making the hair smoother by closing the cuticle scales. Acids are often used as conditioners in shampoos, and as conditioning rinses after alkaline treatments such as perming, bleaching and tinting.

Alkalis

Alkalis are, in general, more damaging to hair than acids. Strong alkalis such as sodium hydroxide at a pH of about 12 are sometimes used in hairdressing preparations to straighten extremely tightly curled hair. Great care is needed with these products. Over-processing could lead to the total destruction of the hair. Strong alkalis with a pH of over 9.5 can burn the skin and act as a depilatory or hair remover. They attack the polypeptide chains in keratin and soften hair until it becomes jelly-like and finally disintegrates.

Less alkaline solutions, such as soap and dilute ammonium hydroxide with a pH of less than 9.5, make hair swell and tend to roughen the cuticle scales (see Fig. 6.10). Ammonium hydroxide (ammonia) is often added to hairdressing preparations to make hair swell to ease the entry of perm lotions, bleaches and dyes into the hair shafts.

Action of salts on the hair

The chemical reaction between an acid and an alkali is called **neutralization** and results in the formation of a salt and water. New substances are always formed during a chemical change and the reaction may be represented by an equation. Neutralization may be represented as follows:

$$\text{An acid} + \text{an alkali} = \text{a salt} + \text{water}$$

Many different salts may be formed by the process of neutralization or by the action of acids on metals. A **salt** always consists of a metal or ammonium radical (from the alkali) and an acid radical (from the acid). Thus ammonium thioglycollate (used in perm lotion) is a salt formed by the chemical reaction between thioglycollic acid and ammonium hydroxide; sodium stearate (a soap) is the salt of stearic acid and sodium

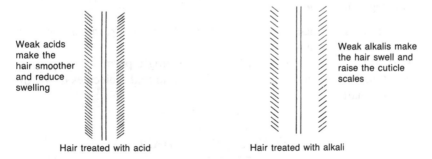

Weak acids make the hair smoother and reduce swelling

Weak alkalis make the hair swell and raise the cuticle scales

Hair treated with acid   Hair treated with alkali

Fig. 6.10 Effect of acids and alkalis on hair

hydroxide; sodium chloride (common salt) is the salt of hydrochloric acid and sodium hydroxide. Salts are usually neutral with a pH of 7 and have little effect on hair condition. A few, such as soap, borax and sodium carbonate (washing soda), are alkaline and if used on hair tend to roughen the cuticle scales and make the hair swell.

Due to their alkalinity, soap shampoos (pH 8−9) are no longer used in salons: neutral or slightly acid soapless shampoos keep the hair in better condition. Ammonium thioglycollate is a salt but is also a reducing agent and is used as a reducing agent in perming.

Neutralization versus neutralizing

Chemical neutralization must not be confused with the process called neutralizing which takes place after cold permanent waving. **Neutralizing** (or normalizing as it is sometimes called) is an oxidation process involving the addition of oxygen and is not the reaction between an acid and alkali.

Action of reducing agents on hair

A **reducing agent** is a substance which will give hydrogen to another substance (or take oxygen away) during a chemical reaction known as **reduction**. Ammonium thioglycollate is a reducing agent used to break some of the cystine linkages in hair during perming. Very strong reducing agents act as depilatories and will destroy hair by breaking both the cystine and peptide linkages in keratin.

Action of oxidizing agents on hair

An **oxidizing agent** is a substance which supplies oxygen (or takes hydrogen away) during a chemical reaction known as **oxidation**. The most common oxidizing agent used in hairdressing is hydrogen peroxide. Hydrogen peroxide

- chemically changes melanin, the natural hair colour, into a colourless compound during bleaching
- rebuilds cystine linkages when neutralizing a perm
- oxidizes permanent dyes to form large coloured molecules inside the hair shaft.

FUNCTIONS OF HAIR

In animals, the main function of hair or fur is to keep the animal warm.

In cold conditions the hairs stand erect, trapping an insulating layer of still air in the fur. Birds fluff out their feathers for the same reason. Human body hairs are insufficient for this purpose, though the hairs do stand erect when the body is cold. Scalp hairs help to keep the head warm, cushion it against blows and protect it from damage by ultra-violet rays in sunlight. However, the main purpose of hair is now one of personal adornment. All hairs are sensitive to touch and increase the sensitivity of the skin to light pressure. The presence of bristly hair is usually protective. The eyebrows prevent sweat from running down the forehead into the eyes, while the lashes prevent the entry of dust. The nostril hairs filter dust from the air as it is breathed in, so cleaning the air before passage to the lungs.

SELF TESTING

1. What pigment is contained (a) in black hair (b) in blonde hair?
2. What is the average diameter of a hair?
3. What is meant by (a) elasticity (b) the elastic limit (c) tensile strength?
4. What gives hair its elastic structure?
5. On what does the porosity of hair depend? Which part of a hair is usually most porous?
6. What is meant by 'hair is hygroscopic'?
7. What properties determine the texture of hair?
8. What is meant by capillary rise?
9. What are the alkaline values on the pH scale?
10. What is the effect on hair of (a) alkalis with a pH of 12 (b) strong acids?
11. Name two organic acids sometimes used as conditioners.
12. What is the difference between chemical neutralization and neutralizing after a permanent wave?
13. Why are soap shampoos no longer used in salons?
14. What are the functions of hair?

7

THE SCALP AND HAIR GROWTH

Scalp hair grows by the division of cells at the base of hair follicles in the skin of the scalp. To enable that growth to take place, nutrients from the food we eat and oxygen from the air we breathe in must be carried through the blood vessels to the dividing cells. The study of the structure of the scalp, skin and hair follicles are necessary for the understanding of hair growth.

STRUCTURE OF THE SCALP

The scalp consists of all the soft tissue covering the bones of the skull from the top of the forehead to the back of the head and to just above the ears at the sides of the head (see Fig. 7.1).

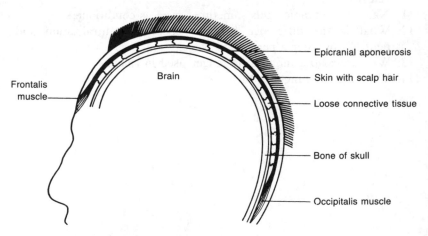

Fig. 7.1 Structure of the scalp

There are two main parts to the scalp

- the **skin** with the scalp hair
- the **epicranial aponeurosis**, which is a broad strong sheet of fibrous tissue or tendon lying under the skin.

The epicranial aponeurosis is firmly attached to the skin by a fatty layer of connective tissue and is also held by frontalis muscle of the forehead and the occipital muscle at the back of the head. Very loose connective tissue attaches the epicranial aponeurosis to the bone of the skull, enabling the whole of the scalp to be moved slightly over the surface of the skull. This movement may be noticed during shampooing. Some people are able to move the epicranial aponeurosis at will by alternately contracting the frontalis and occipital muscles.

STRUCTURE OF THE SKIN

The skin (see Fig. 7.2) consists of two main layers

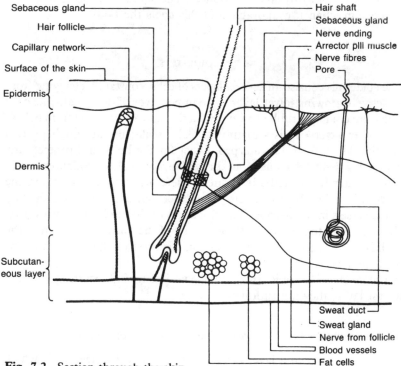

Fig. 7.2 Section through the skin

- the **epidermis** or outer layer
- the **dermis** or true skin forming the inner layer.

Beneath the dermis is the fatty subcutaneous layer which firmly attaches the skin to the epicranial aponeurosis tendon. The boundary between the epidermis and the dermis is clearly defined, but the dermis merges gradually with the subcutaneous layer. Varying amounts of fat stored in the subcutaneous tissue act as insulation to prevent loss of body heat.

The surface of the skin and hair is coated with the slightly acid secretions from two types of glands in the skin, the sebaceous glands and sweat glands. The coating is referred to as the skin's **acid mantle** and has a pH of between 4.5 and 6.

- **Sebaceous glands** open into the hair follicles and secrete an oily substance called sebum which lubricates the skin and hair shafts so helping to make them waterproof. Sebum gives lustre to the hair, though excess makes the hair greasy.
- **Sweat glands** are coiled tubes lying in the dermis with a duct leading to an opening or pore on the surface of the skin. Sweat consists of about 98 per cent water and 2 per cent sodium chloride (common salt) with traces of many other substances. The liquid sweat takes heat from the skin when it evaporates and this cools the body.

The epidermis

The epidermis consists of several layers of cells, constantly changing from an actively growing lower layer to an upper layer of dead scale-like cells which are gradually rubbed away by friction and are replaced from below. The outer layer consists mainly of flaky scales of the tough protein keratin, which forms a waterproof coat for the body and protects the underlying tissue from infection, dirt and injury. It also prevents excessive loss of water from the body tissues. There are very few nerves in the epidermis and no blood vessels. The lower living layer is nourished by blood vessels in the dermis. The thickness of the epidermis varies from about 0.1 mm to 2 mm in different parts of the body, being thin in the eyelids and abdomen, and thickest on the soles of the feet and palms of the hands.

The layers of the epidermis are shown in Fig. 7.3. Starting with the lowest layer, they are as follows:

The germinating layer or basal layer (Stratum germinativum)

This actively growing layer consists of regularly arranged cells which are constantly dividing to form new cells, so pushing the old cells towards

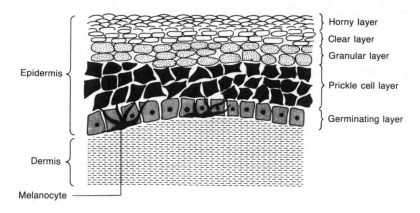

Fig. 7.3 Structure of the epidermis

the surface of the skin. The germinating layer is continuous round the hair follicles, sebaceous glands and sweat glands, and although these structures may appear to be part of the dermis, they are all down growths of the epidermis. Among the cells of this layer are smaller cells called **melanocytes**, which produce the pigment of the skin in the form of yellow, brown or black granules of melanin. Sunbathing increases the production of melanin which protects the skin from damage by the sun's rays, the dark pigment absorbing harmful radiations. Excessive sunbathing, especially by fair skinned people who have little protective melanin, may lead to skin damage and possible cancer.

The prickle cell layer (Stratum spinosum)

This is also known at the Stratum aculeatum. Some of the soft, nucleated cells of this layer have a spiny outgrowth through which it is thought that melanin granules enter the cells. Together with the germinating layer, it forms the living part of the epidermis or **Malpighian layer**.

The granular layer (Stratum granulosum)

The nuclei of the cells in this layer are breaking down, leading to the death of the cells. Keratin is being formed in the cells.

The clear layer (Stratum lucidum)

The flattened cells of this layer contain keratin and have no nuclei. Melanin granules are destroyed in the cells.

The horny layer (Stratum corneum)

The outer layer consists of flat dead cells of keratin which are gradually shed from the surface of the skin by friction, as for example when scales are removed from the scalp during brushing.

The dermis

The dermis joins the epidermis in a series of ridges called **dermal papillae** which are shallow in the scalp. The papillae are well supplied with blood vessels which take nourishment to the growing cells of the epidermis. The blood vessels also help to keep body temperature constant by dilating if the body is too hot and constricting if the body is too cold.

The dermis is between 1 and 4 mm in thickness and consists of a dense network of fibres embedded in a jelly-like ground substance. Many of the fibres are elastic fibres and give the skin flexibility. The ground substance holds a lot of water which makes the skin turgid (firm).

Nerve endings of several types are found in the dermis, making the skin sensitive to pain, heat, cold and pressure. A collar of nerves surrounds each hair follicle (see Fig. 7.2) so hairs are sensitive to touch, and pain is felt if a hair is plucked. These sensations are carried along nerves to the brain.

SELF TESTING

1. Name the broad sheet of tendon in the scalp.
2. How is this tendon connected to the surrounding structures?
3. Name the two main layers of the skin.
4. What is the purpose of subcutaneous fat?
5. What is meant by the acid mantle of the skin? What is the pH value of this mantle?
6. Name the oily secretion of the sebaceous glands. How does the oil affect the hair and skin?
7. Name the five layers of cells in the epidermis. Describe the changes in these cells as they move through the epidermis to the surface of the skin.
8. Name the cells which produce the pigment of the skin. In which layer of the skin are these cells situated?

STRUCTURE OF A HAIR FOLLICLE

A hair follicle (see Fig. 7.4) is formed by the downgrowth of the epidermis into the dermis, the outside of the follicle being a continuation of the germinating layer of the epidermis. The walls of the follicle are known as the **outer root sheath**. The dermis forms a protective sheath of connective tissue round each follicle and also projects upwards into the base of the follicle forming the **hair papilla**. The hair grows from the epidermal cells surrounding the papilla, the cells being nourished from the blood vessels which enter the papilla.

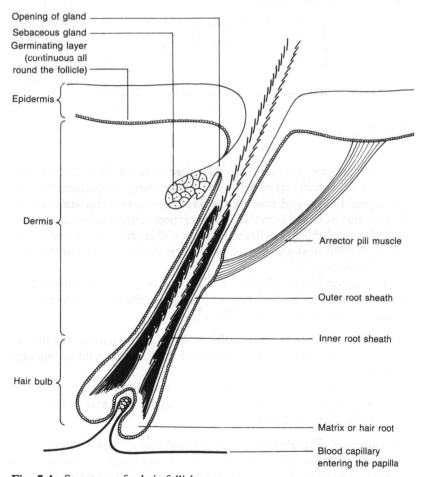

Fig. 7.4   Structure of a hair follicle

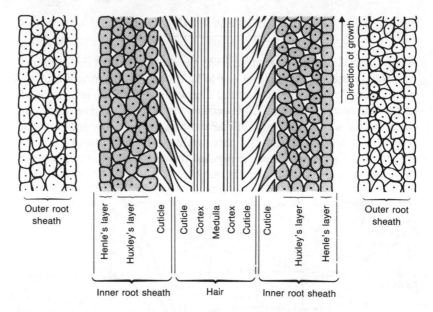

Fig. 7.5 Inner root sheath

A small muscle, the **arrector pili muscle**, is attached to each hair follicle. Cold conditions or fear cause this muscle to contract, moving the sloping follicle and making the hair stand erect, and also making the skin rise in a goose-pimple. The erection of the hair is an attempt by the body to trap an insulating layer of still air between the hairs and skin to prevent heat loss by the body. It is ineffective in humans due to lack of body hair.

While in the follicle, the hair itself is surrounded and protected by the **inner root sheath** which grows up alongside the hair. The inner root sheath consists of three layers (see Fig. 7.5)

- **a cuticle** with overlapping scales pointing to the base of the follicle and so interlocking with the cuticle of the hair and holding the hair firmly
- **Huxley's layer** of two or three cells thickness
- **Henle's layer** of one cell in thickness, which lies next to but separate from the outer root sheath.

The surface of Henle's layer is smooth and able to slip easily over the outer root sheath as the hair and its inner root sheath move upwards together. The inner root sheath breaks down about two-thirds of the way up the follicle at the level of the opening of the sebaceous glands. The passage of the hair along the remaining part of the follicle is eased by the presence of sebum. If a hair is pulled from the scalp, the inner root sheath is removed at the same time and can be seen as a white thickening at the end of the hair.

GROWTH OF HAIR

Hair, like all living material, grows by the division of cells. Each cell is a microscopic unit of living matter consisting of a jelly-like mass, the cytoplasm, surrounded by a membrane through which nourishment can pass into the cell, and through which waste products can leave the cell. A nucleus, usually at the centre of the cell, controls its activity. Groups of cells form tissues such as skin tissue and nerve tissue.

A sample of cells may easily be obtained by scraping the inside of the cheek with a clean spoon or spatula. Place the sample in a drop of water on a slide and cover. Irrigate with iodine by drawing a drop of iodine solution under the cover-slip using blotting paper. Examination under a microscope shows flat pavement cells which form a smooth lining for the cheek (see Fig. 7.6).

New cells are produced when one cell splits into two parts (see Fig. 7.7). The nucleus divides first, followed by the cytoplasm. The division of cells at the base of the hair follicle produces new cells for hair growth. The lower part of the follicle widens out into the hair bulb (see Fig. 7.8).

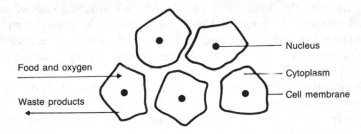

Fig. 7.6 Cell structure

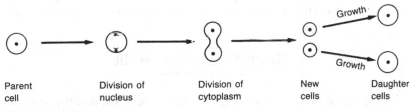

Fig. 7.7 Cell division

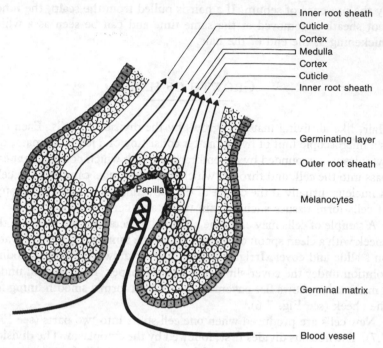

Inner root sheath
Cuticle
Cortex
Medulla
Cortex
Cuticle
Inner root sheath

Germinating layer

Outer root sheath

Melanocytes

Papilla

Germinal matrix

Blood vessel

Fig. 7.8 Hair bulb

This fits over the dermal hair papilla, which contains a knot of small blood vessels. The epidermal cells surrounding the papilla form the germinal matrix or root of the hair. Division of these cells of the epidermis results in hair growth. As new cells are produced they push the older ones upwards.

At first all the cells are alike but as they move up the follicle they begin to change shape, and keratin develops in the cells. The different types of cell for the cuticle, cortex and medulla of the hair and the cells of the inner root sheath develop. By the time they are about one-third of the way up the follicle the cells are dead and fully keratinized. Between the cells surrounding the papilla are melanocytes producing melanin, the pigment of the hair, most of which passes into the cortex of the hair.

NOURISHMENT OF HAIR

The materials required for the growth and development of the new cells are brought to the papilla by the blood. These materials include the products of digestion from the food we eat and oxygen from the air we breathe in. Cells require energy to enable various chemical reactions to take place inside the cells during cell division. Energy is produced when oxygen reacts with glucose from the digestion of carbohydrate foods (sugars and starches). The chemical reaction is an oxidation process as it involves the addition of oxygen to the glucose.

$$\text{Glucose} + \text{oxygen} \rightarrow \text{carbon dioxide} + \text{water} + \text{energy}$$

Mature hair consists mainly of the protein keratin which, like other proteins, is built up from smaller units called amino acids. During digestion, protein foods such as meat, eggs, fish and milk are broken down into amino acids. These are circulated in the bloodstream, sorted and rearranged to build up keratin in the cells of the hair.

BLOOD SUPPLY TO HEAD

Oxygen and the products of digestion of food reach the hair follicles by the circulation of the blood (see Fig. 7.9). Oxygen is carried by haemoglobin in red blood cells, and the products of digestion are dissolved in the liquid part of blood or blood plasma. The heart acts as a pump to circulate blood round the body through the blood vessels.

Oxygenated blood is taken to the head by the **carotid arteries**, which run up through the neck on either side of the windpipe. The internal carotid arteries branch off to pass through the bone of the skull and take blood to the brain. The external carotid arteries remain outside the skull and continue one along each side of the head, branching to supply the muscles and skin of the face and scalp. The branches of the carotid artery are shown in Fig. 7.10. The temporal branch takes blood to the scalp. It divides into very fine blood vessels called capillaries in the skin of the scalp. A small knot of capillaries enters each hair papilla. The capillaries rejoin to form the **jugular veins** which take de-oxygenated blood and waste products back to the heart as shown in Fig. 7.11.

BLOOD SUPPLY TO HAIR PAPILLA

As blood passes through the capillary network in the hair papilla, a liquid oozes out through the porous walls of the capillaries to bathe the surrounding cells. The liquid is **tissue fluid** and is similar to blood plasma. Oxygen which is released from the haemoglobin of red blood cells and the products of digestion (amino acids, fatty acids and glucose)

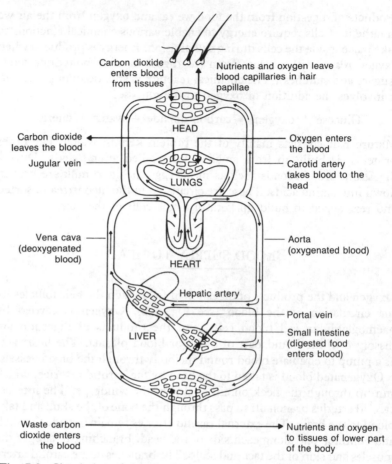

Carbon dioxide enters blood from tissues

Nutrients and oxygen leave blood capillaries in hair papillae

HEAD

Carbon dioxide leaves the blood

Jugular vein

Oxygen enters the blood

Carotid artery takes blood to the head

LUNGS

Vena cava (deoxygenated blood)

Aorta (oxygenated blood)

HEART

Hepatic artery

Portal vein

Small intestine (digested food enters blood)

LIVER

Waste carbon dioxide enters the blood

Nutrients and oxygen to tissues of lower part of the body

Fig. 7.9 Circulation of the blood

are carried by tissue fluid to the cells round the hair papilla, so enabling growth of new hair to take place (see Fig. 7.12). Some of the tissue fluid re-enters the capillaries carrying waste carbon dioxide and some flows away into other channels called **lymph vessels**. This exchange of gases in the tissues is known as **tissue respiration** or **internal respiration**.

The growing hair receives nourishment only through the blood stream. Substances applied externally to the hair shaft do not supply nourishment as the hair cells are then dead and fully keratinized. These substances may, of course, improve the condition of the hair. The nutrition of hair thus depends on diet and the circulation of blood to the scalp. The circulation may be improved by massage. This is often carried out in a salon using hand massage or by use of a vibro massage machine.

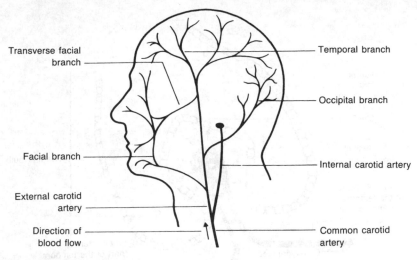

Fig. 7.10   Carotid artery

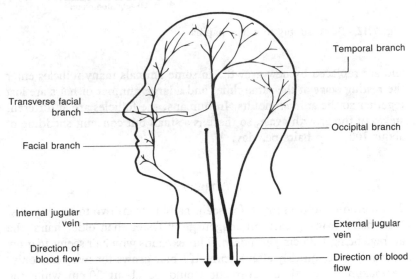

Fig. 7.11   Jugular vein

GROWTH CYCLE OF HAIR

The growth of hair from a particular follicle is not continuous: hair follicles undergo alternate periods of activity (known as **anagen**) and periods of rest (**telogen**). A period of change between activity and rest is known as **catagen** (see Fig. 7.13). During the cycle old hairs are shed

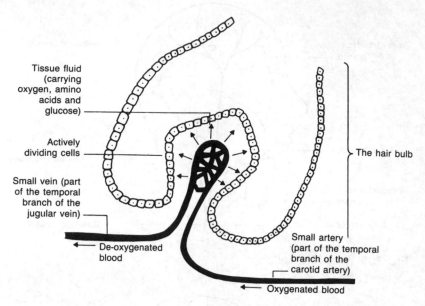

Fig. 7.12 Blood supply to a hair papilla

and are replaced by new growth. In some animals many follicles enter the resting stage at the same time, and a large number of hairs are lost together so the animal moults. In humans, the follicles are at different stages of the growth cycle, so there is a small but constant shedding of about 100 scalp hairs per day.

Anagen

The period of active growth for scalp hairs is from two to seven years. New hairs growing early in anagen grow faster than older hairs, the average being 1.25 cm per month. This explains why hair seems to grow unevenly quite quickly after a trim. If a hair grows for two years only, its maximum length if never cut would be about 30 cm while the maximum length of hair in a seven year cycle is about a metre. Between 80 and 90 per cent of hairs are in anagen at any one time.

Catagen

The period of growth is followed by a short period of change (catagen) before the follicle enters its resting stage. Catagen lasts for about two

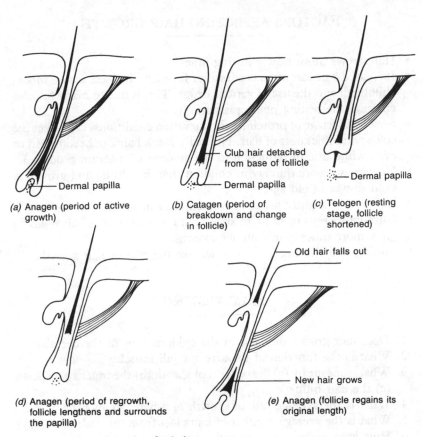

(a) Anagen (period of active growth)

(b) Catagen (period of breakdown and change in follicle)
— Club hair detached from base of follicle
— Dermal papilla

(c) Telogen (resting stage, follicle shortened)
— Dermal papilla

— Dermal papilla

(d) Anagen (period of regrowth, follicle lengthens and surrounds the papilla)

— Old hair falls out

— New hair grows

(e) Anagen (follicle regains its original length)

Fig. 7.13 Growth cycle of a hair

weeks during which activity stops and so new cells are formed. The hair becomes detached from the base of the follicle to form a **club hair**. The hair bulb begins to break down and the follicle becomes shorter by about one-third. At any one time only about 1 per cent of follicles are in catagen.

Telogen

The follicle then enters a resting stage (telogen) for three to four months. About 13 per cent of follicles are in telogen at any one time. When the resting stage is complete the follicle begins to lengthen and a new bulb forms round the cells of the original papilla. When the follicle reaches full length a new hair begins to grow. If the old hair is still in the follicle it is pushed out by the new hair.

FACTORS AFFECTING HAIR GROWTH

- Hair grows more slowly during illness.
- Increased hair loss often occurs after feverish illnesses, severe shock, childbirth and the use of various drugs. This is due to many follicles entering the resting phase prematurely.
- Serious shortage of protein, as in starvation conditions, can affect the colour and thickness of hair. Normally black hair can become red or even white due to reduction in the amount of melanin produced.
- Hair grows more quickly in children than in adults, and growth is even slower in old age.
- Hair grows slightly faster in women than in men.
- Ultra-violet rays in sunlight speed cell division so that hair tends to grow more quickly in summer months.
- Cutting and shaving have no effect on the rate of hair growth.

SELF TESTING

1. Does hair grow from cells of the epidermis or of the dermis?
2. What is the function of the arrector pili muscle?
3. What is meant by (a) the outer root sheath (b) the inner root sheath (c) the hair bulb?
4. What is the average rate of growth of a hair per month?
5. What is the average number of hairs lost from the scalp each day?
6. How long is the period of active growth of a hair (anagen)?
7. What is meant by a club hair?
8. What is the name given to the resting period of a follicle?
9. How long is a follicle usually in the resting stage?
10. What factors affect hair growth?
11. What are the main materials needed for hair growth?
12. How do these materials reach the hair follicles?

PART 3

CONSULTATION AND DIAGNOSIS

8

DISORDERS OF THE SCALP AND HAIR

During the course of their work hairdressers will inevitably encounter clients with various infections, non-infectious conditions and infestations of the hair and scalp. Hairdressers should be able to recognize common diseases and conditions, so that they can judge the advisability of carrying out various hairdressing processes.

The scalp and hair should be examined before any treatment is given. If infectious conditions or infestations are noticed no further service should be offered. The client must be advised tactfully and sympathetically that salon treatment cannot continue and medical advice should be sought. Any equipment used on the client must be cleaned and sterilized before re-use. Where non-infectious conditions are present, normal hairdressing services can usually be carried out and in some cases conditioning treatments or special shampoos may be recommended as being beneficial.

INFECTIOUS CONDITIONS

An infectious disease is one which can be passed from one person to another by either direct contact with an infected person or indirectly from an infected object. Infection itself is caused by the presence of micro-organisms which may be classified as fungi, bacteria and viruses.

Tinea capitis (ringworm of the scalp)

Causative organism: Fungus which grows into the epidermis of the skin and invades hair and follicles (see Fig. 8.1 and refer back to Fig. 3.1).

Occurrence: Mostly in children under 12. After that age the

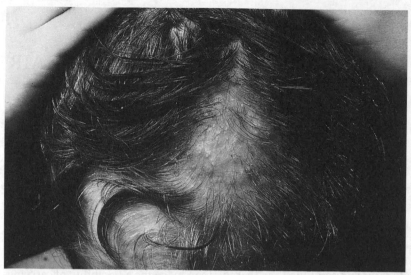

Fig. 8.1 Ringworm of the scalp

	production of sebum, which is slightly fungicidal, increases and protects the skin from infection.
Signs of disease:	Round patches of greyish scaly skin on the scalp with short stubbly broken-off hairs.
Method of spread:	By direct contact with an infected head or by indirect contact with broken-off infected hairs in brushes, combs or towels.
Treatment:	Ringworm is highly infectious. No hairdressing service must be given. No salon treatment for the condition is possible. Medical treatment is required.

Impetigo

Causative organism:	Bacteria which enter breaks in the skin (see Fig. 8.2).
Occurrence:	Mostly in children on the face or scalp or in the beard area of men. May follow infestation by head lice.
Signs of disease:	Small blisters on the skin filled with a clear liquid which may ooze or weep. Later followed by yellow crusts.
Method of spread:	By touching the infected area or by infected towels but the infection must enter a break in the skin.

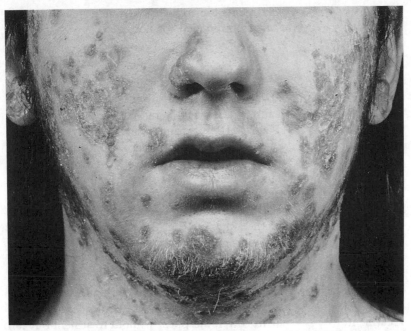

Fig. 8.2 Impetigo

	May lead to folliculitis.
Treatment:	Impetigo is highly infectious.
	No hairdressing service must be given.
	No salon treatment for the condition is possible.
	Medical treatment is required.

Folliculitis

Causative organism:	Bacteria which enter hair follicles.
Occurrence:	May occur on the scalp or in the beard area in men. Sometimes follows impetigo.
Signs of disease:	Small yellow pustules with a hair in the centre.
Method of spread:	By direct contact with an infected person (touch) or by a scratch from an infected tool. Irritation due to 'pull burns' during perming, in which perm lotion enters the follicles, may lead to scratching followed by folliculitis.
Treatment:	If widespread, no hairdressing service must be given.
	No salon treatment for the condition is possible.
	Medical treatment is recommended. Antibiotic

ointments are applied. Cetrimide shampoos may be recommended for home use.

Warts (verrucae)

Causative organism:
: Viruses living in the lower layer of the epidermis causing abnormal keratinization to take place.

Occurrence:
: Plane warts occur mostly in children on the backs of the hands or on the face round the hair line. Common warts occur at any age but mostly in children and young adults, usually on the hands or face.

Signs of disease:
: Flesh-coloured growths raised above the surface of the skin (see Fig. 8.3). May be small, round and numerous with a smooth flat top (plane or juvenile warts), or larger and rough-topped (common warts).

Method of spread:
: By touch, though they are not highly contagious. Direct contact with warts should be avoided.

Treatment:
: Warts often disappear without treatment but can be removed by a doctor. Removal of warts from a hairdresser's hands is advised as they are

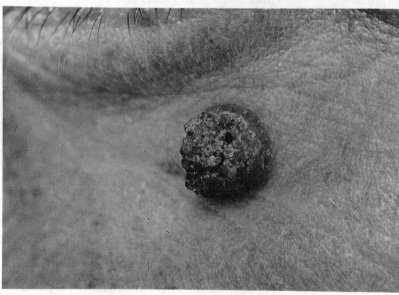

Fig. 8.3 Common wart

unsightly as well as infectious and clients may object to them.

Warts themselves cannot be treated in a salon. Normal hairdressing services can be carried out but care should be taken not to damage warts.

INFESTATION BY PARASITES

A **parasite** is a living creature which obtains its food supply by living on or in the body of another living organism known as the **host**. The presence of small animal parasites on the skin is called an **infestation**. This is not an infection in itself, but may lead to secondary infection such as boils or impetigo, if bacteria enter breaks in the skin caused either by the bites of the parasite or scratching by the host in an attempt to relieve itching.

Pediculosis capitis (infestation by head lice)

Head lice (see Fig. 8.4) are small, light brown or grey insects usually found in the hair at the back of the head but in severe cases may have spread to other areas as well. The adult female is about 2–3 mm long

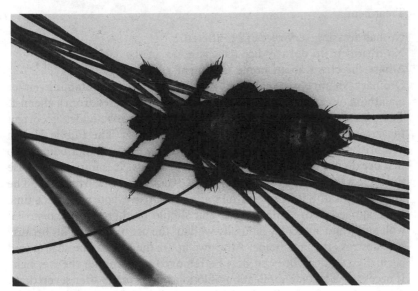

Fig. 8.4 Head louse in hair

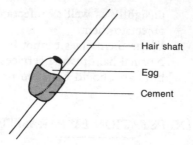

Fig. 8.5   Nit attached to a hair

and 1 mm wide; the male is slightly smaller. The louse (**pediculus capitis**) has six legs each ending in a claw enabling it to cling to the hair shafts. It feeds by piercing the skin of the host and drawing blood. The female lays about 300 eggs, called **nits** (see Fig. 8.5), in a life of 4–5 weeks. The nits are white and shiny, and are oval in shape. A gummy cement firmly attaches the nits to the hair, usually close to the scalp. The eggs take about a week to hatch and the young a week to mature. They are then capable of reproducing themselves.

Lice are most common in children. They are easily passed from person to person by direct contact or by infested objects such as brushes, combs, towels or gowns. Any equipment used on a client with lice should be sterilized and gowns, towels, etc., washed immediately.

Treatment

No hairdressing service can be offered.
No treatment to destroy lice can be given in the salon.
Advise the client about home treatment as follows:
Ordinary shampooing will not kill lice. A lotion containing either **malathion** or **carbaryl** as an insecticide can be purchased from a chemist. The pharmacist should know which of the two insecticides is correct for current use in the area where the client lives. The Public Health authorities recommend alternate use of the two lotions periodically so that lice do not become resistant to the chemicals. It is important to use the correct lotion if infestation by lice is eventually to be overcome. The lotions will kill both lice and nits after about two hours' contact time when applied to dry hair. All the hair should be thoroughly moistened with lotion and left to dry naturally without the use of a hair dryer because heat destroys the insecticide. After two hours the hair can be shampooed normally and dead lice can best be removed by combing the wet hair. If necessary a second application of lotion can be made after seven days. All members of a family should be treated at the same time.

SELF TESTING

1. Name three infectious conditions affecting the scalp, stating in each case the micro-organism responsible for the condition.
2. Which conditions would appear on the scalp as:
   (a) small yellow pustules with a hair in the centre?
   (b) a scaly patch with broken-off hairs?
3. By what signs would you recognize impetigo? How is impetigo spread?
4. How may ringworm be spread from person to person?
5. What is the difference in appearance between plane warts and common warts? How may warts be spread?
6. What is meant by (a) a parasite (b) an infestation?
7. Describe and name the eggs of a louse.
8. How and where are the eggs attached to hair?
9. How does a louse obtain nourishment?
10. What advice would you offer to a client with head lice?
11. Name two insecticides used in lotions to kill lice.

NON-INFECTIOUS CONDITIONS

Psoriasis

Appearance: Thick patches of silvery scales on the scalp (see Fig. 8.6). Under the scales, the skin may be red and bleeding may occur if the scales are removed.

Cause: Abnormal formation of keratin in skin cells. The condition is thought to be inherited and often affects several members of the same family. It may also be stress related and often clears, returning again in times of stress.

Treatment: Normal hairdressing services can be carried out. Use minimum of massage during shampooing to avoid stimulation of cell division which builds up the scales. **Coal tar shampoos** are useful but medical treatment is more effective.

Pityriasis capitis (dandruff)

Appearance: Patches of small, dry, itchy scales on the scalp. In severe cases, grey or white scales constantly fall from the scalp.

Cause: Overactive production and shedding of epidermal scales.

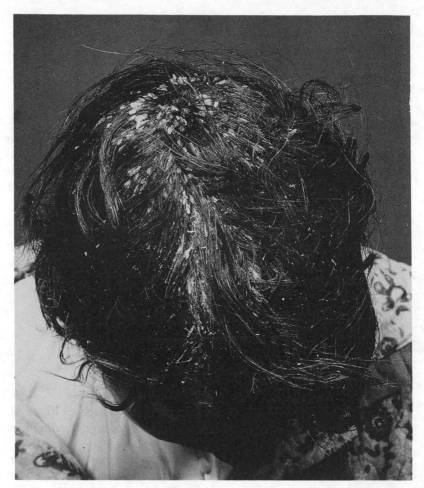

Fig. 8.6 Psoriasis

Treatment: Anti-dandruff shampoos containing **keratolytics** (keratin splitters) such as **zinc pyrithione** (zinc omadine), which is also an antiseptic, are effective. **Selenium sulphide** is sometimes used but may cause dermatitis. Dandruff provides a breeding ground for bacteria and yeast cells, and so medicated shampoos containing cetrimide or hexachlorophane are useful but do not clear dandruff. Dandruff is often treated at home.

Normal hairdressing services can be carried out. Oil conditioning treatments are beneficial. If the condition is very severe, medical advice is required.

Alopecia

Alopecia is a general term meaning baldness. There are many different types.

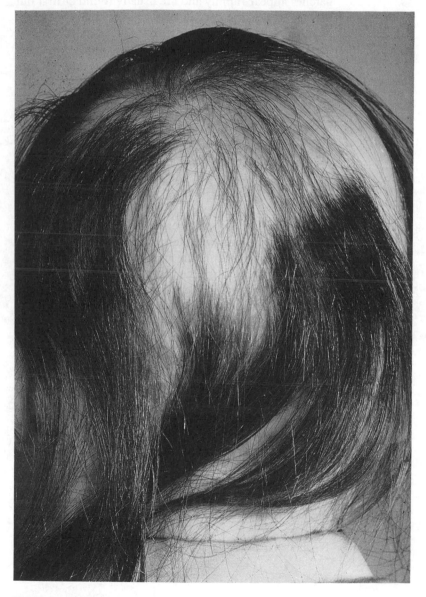

Fig. 8.7 Alopecia arcata

Alopecia areata

Appearance: Small bald patches on the scalp sometimes following the line of a nerve (see Fig. 8.7). The area is completely bald with no broken-off hairs as seen in ringworm. The bald patches appear rapidly and are usually round at first but may be oval if the condition spreads. Patches may join together to form larger areas of baldness.

Cause: Nervous origin. Follows stress or shock. Possible hereditary tendency.

Treatment: Regrowth often takes place after two to three months without treatment, but the condition may recur in times of stress.
Normal hairdressing services can be carried out. Salon high frequency treatment or massage may be beneficial. Medical treatment is advisable.

Cicatrical alopecia

Appearance: Irregularly shaped permanently bald area.

Cause: Damage to the skin with destruction of the follicles and the formation of scar tissue after severe cuts or burns by heat or chemicals, e.g. incorrect use of sodium hydroxide in hair straightening if the lotion comes into contact with the skin. Burns due to a hot blow dryer touching the skin.

Treatment: None. The follicles have been destroyed, therefore regrowth cannot take place.
Normal hairdressing services can be carried out.

Male pattern baldness (androgenic alopecia)

Appearance: Symmetrical hair loss starting at the front margins with hair gradually receding at the temples (see Figs 8.8a and 8.8b). Thinning may also occur at the crown. The two areas may join to leave a fringe of hair over the ears and at the back of the head.

Cause: A sex-linked hereditary condition.

Treatment: Medical treatments are being developed. Hair transplants are possible.
Normal hairdressing services can be carried out.

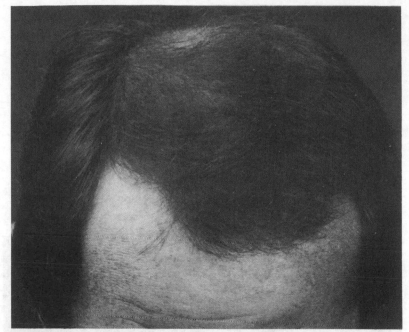

Fig. 8.8a   Male pattern baldness (early)

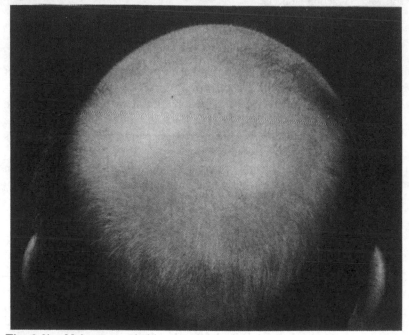

Fig. 8.8b   Male pattern baldness (advanced)

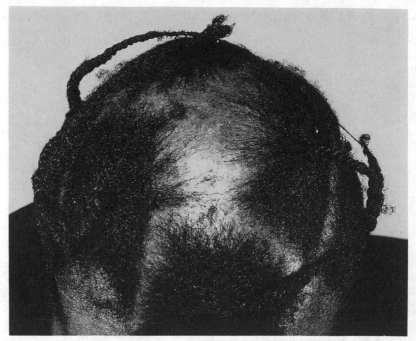

Fig. 8.9 Traction alopecia

Traction alopecia

Appearance: Baldness at any part of scalp where hair has been subject to repeated traction or pulling (see Fig. 8.9).

Cause: Frequent traction or pulling of the hair shafts, for example constantly pulling hair back in a pony tail or bun causes hair loss at the front margins; tight plaiting causes loss at the base of the plait.

Treatment: None. Hair may regrow if traction is discontinued but in some cases the baldness may be permanent.
Normal hairdressing services can be carried out.

DISORDERS OF THE SEBACEOUS GLANDS (NON-INFECTIOUS)

Seborrhoea

Appearance: Lank, greasy hair. Greasy areas of skin especially round the nose and on the forehead.

Cause: Overactivity of sebaceous glands producing excess sebum.

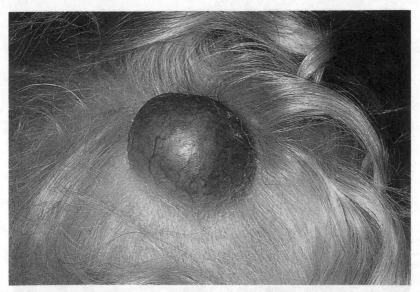

Fig. 8.10   Sebaceous cyst

Treatment: Regular shampooing using shampoos designed for greasy hair but avoiding too much brushing or massage, which stimulates sebum production. Avoid the use of oily products. Alkaline rinses of weak solutions of borax help to remove grease. Spirit lotions may be useful to reduce sebum production.

Normal hairdressing services can be carried out.

Sebaceous cyst

Appearance: The cyst forms a lump under the surface of the skin of the scalp (see Fig. 8.10). The size varies from pea-sized to the size of an egg. The surface of the cyst may be devoid of hair. Sometimes an unpleasant-smelling fatty material may be squeezed from the cyst.

Cause: Blockage of the sebaceous gland.

Treatment: Cysts cannot be removed in a salon and care is needed not to damage the skin over the cyst when brushing or combing the hair.

Normal hairdressing services can be carried out. Cysts can be removed surgically if desired but are often left untreated.

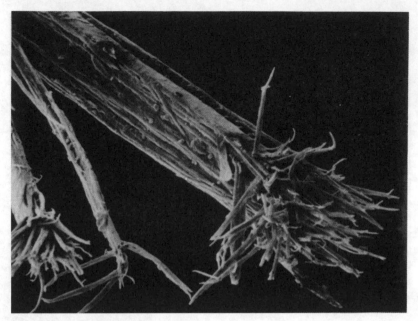

Fig. 8.11   Fragilitas crinium

DISORDERS OF THE HAIR SHAFT (NON-INFECTIOUS)

Fragilitas crinium (split ends)

Appearance: Dry, brittle hair, split lengthways at the ends and possibly at other places along the shaft (see Fig. 8.11). Often occurs in long hair.

Cause: Physical or chemical damage. Daily brushing and combing, shampooing and periodic perming, tinting or bleaching over a number of years and over-exposure to sun and wind.

Treatment: Best treated by cutting off split ends and reconditioning the remainder by protein-based substantive conditioners, restructurants or conditioners containing silicone oils which tend to 'glue' the ends together.

Trichorrhexis nodosa

Appearance: Nodes or small split swellings on the hair shaft (see Fig. 8.12). The hair may break off at the nodes.

Cause: Physical or chemical damage, such as use of spiked rollers,

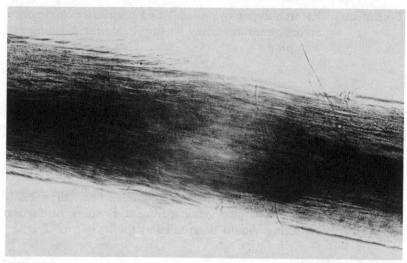

Fig. 8.12   Trichorrhexis nodosa

tight rubbers during perming, severe back combing or chemically by use of too strong perm lotions or bleaches. Seasonally in late summer due to over-exposure to sun.

Treatment: Reconditioning by protein-based substantive conditioners or restructurants. Damaged hair may not be suitable for perming and bleaching. Avoid the use of heated rollers and hot brushes.

Damaged cuticle

Appearance: Dull, rough hair.
Cause: Physical damage or chemical over-processing or weathering.

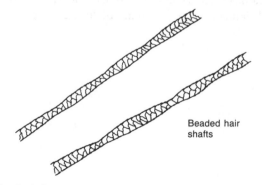

Beaded hair
shafts

Fig. 8.13   Monilethrix

Treatment: Reconditioning by protein-based substantive conditioners or restructurants. May be unsuitable for perming and bleaching.

Monilethrix

Appearance: A beaded hair shaft in which the thickness of the hair varies along its length (see Fig. 8.13). Hair tends to break off easily and is usually very short.

Cause: A rare hereditary condition resulting in uneven keratin production in the follicle.

Treatment: Gentle massage with vegetable oils. The hair is easily broken so requires gentle treatment. Perming, tinting and bleaching should be avoided as the hair is too fragile.

SELF TESTING

1. Which non-infectious conditions may be caused by stress?
2. Which non-infectious conditions may require medical attention?
3. How would you know the difference between patches of alopecia areata and a case of ringworm?
4. How do the scales of dandruff differ from those of psoriasis?
5. Name two ingredients of anti-dandruff shampoos.
6. Which non-infectious conditions are regarded as being hereditary?
7. What are the causes of (a) trichorrhexis nodosa (b) sebaceous cysts?
8. How may the following conditions be treated in the salon:
   (a) seborrhoea (b) fragilitas crinium (c) damaged cuticle?
9. Name a non-infectious condition caused by uneven production of keratin in a growing hair.
10. Which non-infectious conditions can be caused by physical or chemical damage (a) to the hair (b) to the scalp?

9

Hair condition

One important aim in hairdressing is to keep the client's hair in the best possible condition. A hairdresser must therefore be able to recognize the signs of good hair condition, and understand the causes and effects of hair damage.

Recognizing hair condition

Hair in good condition

- feels soft and pliable
- is smooth to the touch and does not tangle easily
- has lustre (shine)
- has high tensile strength so does not break easily
- has high elasticity
- is manageable, easy to brush and comb, and easy to set.

Hair in poor condition

Hair in poor condition may reveal one or more of the following problems: it may

- be lank and greasy
- look dull and uninteresting
- feel dry or very dry, with split ends or splits in the hair shaft and be easily tangled
- be porous and absorb water or other liquids readily
- lack elasticity so giving a poor set
- be easily broken.

Surface and internal effect

Hair condition depends on a **surface effect** due to the state of the cuticle and degree of oiliness of the surface scales and an **internal effect** depending on the state of the chemical linkages inside the hair and the amount of moisture in the hair shaft.

SURFACE CONDITION

When in good condition, the cuticle scales lie flat and close together, giving a relatively smooth surface. In damaged hair some of the scales may be raised, the surface worn away, and the edges of the scales chipped (see Fig. 9.1). In severely damaged hair, cuticle scales may be completely destroyed thus exposing the cortex and possibly leading to the splitting of the hair shaft. Hair with a damaged cuticle feels rough to the touch and is more porous.

The roughness of hair, especially if it is dry, often leads to the production of static electricity when the hair is brushed or combed (refer back to Fig. 5.2).

Roughness of the surface also leads to a dull appearance. A smooth hair reflects light regularly, so that most of the light leaves the surface at the same angle giving the surface lustre or gloss (see Fig. 9.2). A rough surface absorbs more light than a smooth surface, and reflects light irregularly. Less light is reflected and the reflected light is diffused or scattered in all directions giving the surface a matt or dull appearance (see Fig. 9.3). A thin coating of oil (sebum or a dressing cream) on the surface of the hair improves smoothness and increases the amount of light which is regularly reflected so adding lustre. A thick coating of oil due to over-secretion of the sebaceous glands, as in seborrhoea, tends to absorb the light and reduce reflection, making the hair dull.

A thin coating of sebum on the cuticle makes the hair more pliable and therefore less brittle. The hair is easier to comb and the danger of cuticle damage by friction is reduced. Sebum also makes the hair more waterproof and decreases porosity. Insufficient secretion of sebum or excessive removal of sebum during shampooing may allow moisture already in the hair shaft to dry out, again leading to poor condition.

Damage to the cuticle makes hair more porous, possibly resulting in increased absorption of chemicals which in turn can cause internal damage to the hair.

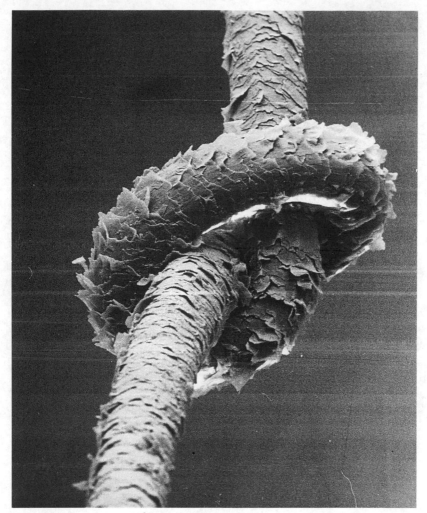

Fig. 9.1 Micro-photograph of a damaged hair

INTERNAL CONDITION

In **virgin hair** (hair which has been untreated by chemicals) the chemical linkages of keratin are intact. Chemical treatments such as perming, tinting and bleaching, particularly if incorrectly carried out, may result in permanent loss of the cross linkages and bonds of the hair. Some parts

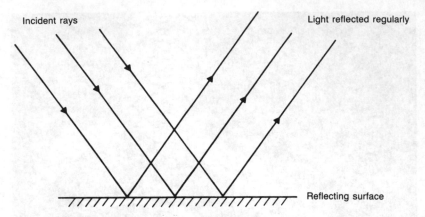

Fig. 9.2   Light reflected from a smooth hair

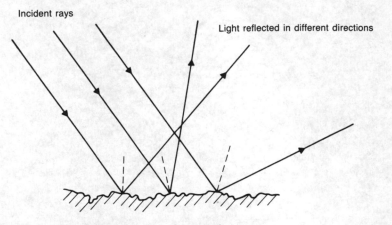

Fig. 9.3   Light reflected from a rough hair

of hair protein may become soluble and be washed from the hair. These losses weaken the hair structure, elasticity may be reduced, and breakage of the hair shaft itself may take place.

Elasticity depends on the coiled spring arrangement of the molecules of hair keratin which gives hair 'bounce', and enables the hair to be stretched and to spring back when tension is released (see Fig. 9.4). The amount of stretching is limited by the numerous hydrogen bonds between the coils of the polypeptide chains and the cystine cross linkages between adjacent chains. Most of the water in the hair shaft is drawn up into the narrow air spaces between the cortical fibres by capillary action. Some is in the form of bound water which extends the hydrogen bonds and

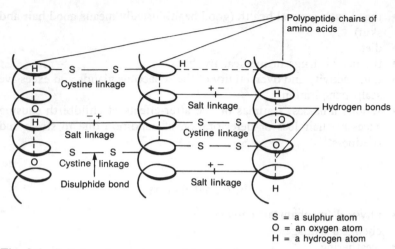

Fig. 9.4 Coiled spring structure of keratin

increases elasticity. If some of the cystine linkages have been lost due to chemical damage, the hair will stretch even further but will not spring back and will not take a good set.

The tensile strength of a hair is a measure of how strong a hair is or how easily it will break. It depends on the strength of the polypeptide chains in keratin and also on the cross linkages holding the chains together. An average hair, if dry, will support a 120–50 gram weight before breaking at its weakest point. The tensile strength of hair is lower when wet and it will break more easily. If the structure of keratin is weakened by chemical action, breakage may occur when tension is applied to the hair, for example tension should be avoided immediately after the application of perm lotion when many cystine linkages are broken.

Moisture in the capillary spaces of the hair affects the thickness of hair. Low moisture content leads to fine lank hair. With a high moisture content the hair swells slightly so adding bulk, and the hair feels soft and pliable. In damaged hair with fewer cross linkages in the cortex, more water can be absorbed and the hair may become waterlogged and difficult to dry out.

CAUSES OF POOR CONDITION

Internal physiological factors

- hereditary conditions affecting the strength and texture of hair

- the client's general health (good health usually means good hair and skin)
- diet
- the use of drugs in medical treatment
- underactivity and overactivity of the sebaceous glands and excessive scalp perspiration
- serious illnesses, traumas or the after-effects of childbirth causing excessive hair loss or deterioration of condition due to stress and tiredness.

External factors

- physical (mechanical) damage
- chemical damage
- weathering.

It is with the external factors that a hairdresser has most control but treatment is still required for poor condition whatever the cause.

PHYSICAL DAMAGE

The cuticle scales can be damaged by any form of friction (rubbing) applied to the hair. The effect is increased if the hair is wet as the cuticle is softened and more easily removed or damaged. An exposed cortex is readily damaged, especially by wet brushing, causing splitting of the hair shaft particularly at the points.

Damage by friction

Damage by friction can be caused during the following activities:

- Excessive massage during shampooing.
- Towel drying: blotting is less damaging than vigorous rubbing.
- Normal brushing and combing, especially by use of an unsuitable brush or a broken comb. Normal grooming always leads to increased damage towards the points of the hair which have been brushed and combed over a longer period. Frontal hair may suffer more damage than other areas of the scalp by more frequent attention.
- Back brushing or combing. Fragments of raised cuticle may be broken off.

- Brushing or combing wet hair as in blow drying. Use of silicone setting lotions will reduce damage.
- Habitually pushing the hair away from the face.
- Normal rubbing of long hair against the shoulders.

Other causes

Other possible causes of physical damage include the following:

- use of spiked rollers or excessively tight rollers
- dreadlocks or the continual wearing of postiche (false hair pieces)
- frequent heat treatment, e.g. hot brushing, crimping, tonging or blow drying
- tension on the hair after application of cold wave lotion
- incorrect razor cutting: 'slithering', a sliding movement of the razor, can strip off sections of the cuticle.

CHEMICAL DAMAGE

Most chemical damage takes place during bleaching, perming and hair straightening and to a lesser extent during tinting.

Damage to the cuticle

Damage to the cuticle is caused by any alkaline treatment including bleaching, perming, hair straightening, tinting and the use of soap shampoos. Alkalis make the hair swell and roughen the cuticle scales. Sections of cuticle often break away during bleaching and perming. Damage can be lessened by the use of **fillers** to even out porosity before treatment and the use of acid-based conditioners after treatment. The scales may also be scorched during blow drying if the hot nozzle touches the hair.

Damage to cystine linkages

Damage to cystine linkages always occurs during perming and bleaching. The aim of perming is to break some of the cystine linkages, mould the hair on curlers to give the desired shape, then rebuild the linkages during neutralizing to hold the hair in its newly curled state. However, some loss of cystine linkages always takes place. Over-processing during perming or insufficient neutralizing increase this loss. During bleaching up to 50 per cent of cystine linkages may be destroyed. Hair damaged by loss of cystine linkages is weakened and suffers loss of elasticity. The hair will stretch but not spring back.

Loss of protein material

Loss of protein material from the hair always takes place during perming and bleaching because soluble products are formed which may be washed out of the hair.

Breakage of the hair shaft

Breakage of the hair shaft due to chemical damage to the polypeptide chains may occur by:

- use of products with a pH greater than 9.5, e.g. too long contact time with sodium hydroxide in hair straightening
- excessive oxidation during bleaching
- use of hydrogen peroxide on hair previously treated with metallic dyes
- perming of damaged hair, e.g. excessively bleached hair
- use of strong reducing agents.

Effect of bleaches

- There is always some damage to the cuticle by alkaline processing and loss of cross linkages by oxidation, especially if bleaching very dark hair to blonde. Damaged protein material may be washed out of the hair. Hair becomes more porous, less elastic and has a lower tensile strength. The hair may become waterlogged and difficult to dry out but straw-like when dry.
- Over-bleaching can lead to splitting of the peptide linkages in the polypeptide chains and result in hair breakage.
- Overlapping during retouching may damage or break off cuticle scales, and may also cause hair breakage.

Effect of perm lotions

- Alkaline perms leave the cuticle rough and the hair dull and porous.

- There is always some loss of cystine linkages which reduces tensile strength.
- Over-processing breaks more cystine linkages than can be repaired during neutralizing and so weakens the hair. Hair breakage may occur.

Effect of neutralizers

- Over-neutralizing changes cystine into cysteic acid which does not form cross linkages. The hair is therefore weakened.
- Under-neutralizing results in the rebuilding of fewer cystine linkages, again weakening the hair.

Effect of tints

Tinting is an alkaline process and so roughens the cuticle and makes the hair more porous.
- Some damage to the cystine linkages may occur if the hydrogen peroxide used is too strong.

Effect of colour reducers (strippers)

Colour reducers are strong reducing agents and if left on the hair too long will act as depilatories, destroying the hair by breaking both cystine and peptide linkages.

WEATHERING

It is difficult to distinguish damage caused by exposure to the weather from that caused chemically or physically by other means.

Effect of weathering

- Exposure to the ultra-violet rays in strong sunlight causes most damage. Cystine linkages are broken, reducing tensile strength and causing the relaxation of curl in perms. Bleaching of both natural hair colour and dyed hair takes place.
- Heat from the sun dries out moisture in the hair, roughens the cuticle and encourages breakages and split ends. At the end of long hot

summers there is often an increase of cases of fragilitas crinium and trichorrhexis nodosa.

- The effect of sunlight is greater if the hair is already damaged by chemical treatment, e.g. bleaching, or is weak and brittle, as in cases of monilethrix.
- Exposure to high winds may cause tangling of the hair with possible damage to the cuticle scales.
- High humidity in the air causes increased absorption of moisture because hair is hygroscopic. This improves elasticity and softness of the hair but also leads to loss of set. Loss of moisture from the hair in conditions of very low humidity leads to dryness and lack of flexibility of hair but sets last much longer.

Sunscreen sprays

Sunscreen sprays, containing para-aminobenzoic acid in a plastic resin-based hair spray, are available to lessen sun damage to hair but a more effective way is to cover the hair and avoid exposure to the sun.

SELF TESTING

1. Describe the 'feel' of hair which is in poor condition.
2. What is meant by (a) tensile strength (b) porous hair?
3. How does the condition of the cuticle affect reflection of light?
4. What is the effect on the hair of (a) a small amount of sebum (b) a thick coating of sebum?
5. What is meant by static electricity and how may it be produced on hair?
6. How does the moisture content of hair affect its condition?
7. What is the chief cause of physical damage to the cuticle?
8. What are the effects of alkaline treatments on the condition of hair?
9. In what ways may the hair suffer damage during blow drying?
10. What type of linkages in hair keratin are damaged during perming and bleaching?
11. What damage may result from perming over-bleached hair?
12. What is meant by weathering?
13. What is the effect on hair of over-exposure to strong sunlight?
14. What is meant by a sunscreen spray and what is the active ingredient?

10

CHOICE OF STYLE AND CHEMICAL PROCESSING

The choice of style and any decision to carry out chemical processing must be made as a result of consultation between client and hairdresser. The possible style may be limited by the client's features, the amount and length of hair, how the hair grows and its general condition. The hairdresser must advise the client after assessing these limitations. If the client desires chemical treatments such as perming, bleaching or permanent colouring, the hairdresser must be certain that the process will not cause serious damage and that a satisfactory result can be obtained. Various tests can be carried out prior to treatment to help in making a decision. The hairdresser may have to suggest to the client that the treatment is unsuitable. This should be done with tact and alternatives suggested.

SUITABILITY OF A STYLE

The suitability of a style depends on

- the shape of the head and face
- facial features and length of neck
- the growth patterns, amount of lift and direction of growth of hair
- the quantity, type and texture of the hair
- hair condition
- the age, lifestyle and personality of the client.

STRUCTURE OF THE HEAD

The shape of the face and head are largely determined by

- the bone structure of the **skull**
- the **muscles** of the head and neck.

The skull

The skull consists of two parts: the **cranium**, which is a protective box holding the brain, and the **face** (see Figs 10.1 and 10.2). There are eight bones in the cranium and fourteen in the face. The only movable bone in the skull is the lower jaw, which is hinged to allow chewing and talking. All the other bones are held rigidly together by saw-edged joints or **sutures**.

Bones of the cranium

The bones of the cranium are as follows:

- **The frontal bone** forms the forehead and the front part of the top of the skull.
- **A pair of parietal bones** join down the mid-line of the top of the skull.
- **The occipital bone** forms the back and part of the base of the skull. In it is a large opening, the foramen magnum, through which passes the spinal cord.
- **A pair of temporal bones** form the lower part of the sides of the cranium and contain cavities for the ear passages. A portion of the temporal bone juts out to join the cheek bone forming the **zygomatic arch** which may be felt just in front of the lower part of the ear. The mastoid process is a projection from the temporal bone forming a small

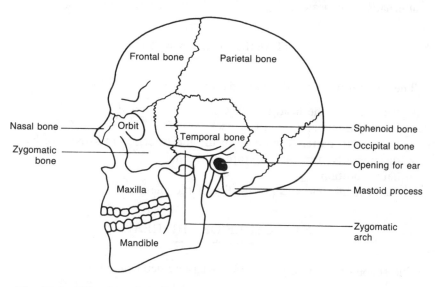

Fig. 10.1   Side view of skull

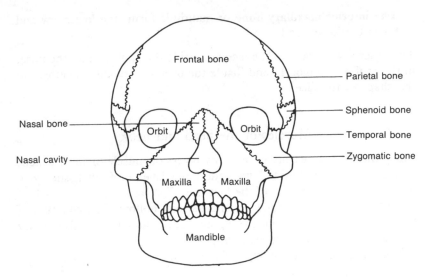

Fig. 10.2 Front view of skull

lump just behind the ear. This surrounds and protects the inner part of the ear and also forms a point of attachment for the sternomastoid muscle in the neck.

- **The sphenoid bone** occupies most of the base of the cranium. It is shaped like a bat with its extended wing tips forming part of each side of the skull between the temporal and frontal bones.
- **The ethmoid bone**, a small irregularly shaped bone, forms part of the base of the cranium, the roof of the nose and inner wall of the **orbits** (eye-sockets). This bone is not shown in the diagrams.

Bones of the face

The following bones give shape to the face:

- **A pair of small nasal bones** make the bridge of the nose. The rest of the nose contains cartilage which is softer and more flexible than bone. This cartilage determines the shape of the tip of the nose.
- **A pair of zygomatic bones** (malar) form the cheek bones which may be felt just below the eyes. The zygomatic arches join the cheek bones and the temporal bones providing a place of attachment for the muscles raising the upper lip.
- **The two superior maxillary bones** or maxillae form the upper jaw and hold the upper teeth.

- **The inferior maxillary bone** or mandible forms the lower jaw and holds the lower teeth.

The other seven bones of the face are inside the skull behind the nose, in the roof of the mouth, and inside the orbits: they have no effect on the shape of the face.

Muscles of the head and neck

The bones of the face are covered by layers of muscle or flesh which, together with the skin and its underlying layer of fatty tissue, give roundness to the contours of the face (see Figs 10.3 and 10.4). Lack of subcutaneous fat may make the cheeks look hollow. The contours of the face change with age due to sagging muscles and decreased elasticity of the skin, causing wrinkles to appear.

There are three main groups of muscles.

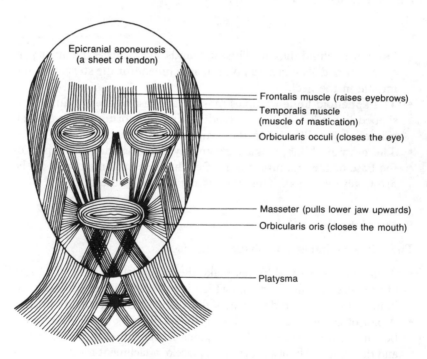

Fig. 10.3 Muscles of the face

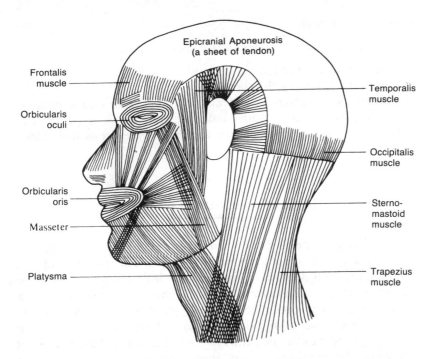

Fig. 10.4 Muscles of the head and neck

Muscles of facial expression

Circular muscles (the orbicularis oculi) surround each eye, enabling it to be screwed up or opened wide. A similar circular muscle (the orbicularis oris) surrounds the mouth for movement of the lips in speaking, pouting, whistling, etc. Groups of small muscles radiate from this circular muscle to raise and lower the angle of the mouth when smiling or looking 'down in the mouth'. Small muscles just above the eyes cause frowning and other muscles wrinkle the nose.

Muscles of mastication

The masseter and the temporalis muscles enable chewing and biting to take place. The temporalis lies over the temporal bone and joins the jaw after passing in front of the ear. The masseter joins the jaw to the zygomatic arch.

Muscles of the neck

There are three main muscles in the neck:

- **The sterno-mastoid** is used in turning the head.
- **The trapezius** raises the shoulders.
- **The platysma** is a thin sheet of muscle just under the skin of the neck. It stretches from the mouth, under the chin and down the neck to the chest. It is used in swallowing and also in the expression of sudden fear.

SHAPE OF THE HEAD AND NECK

The variation of head shape in different people is due largely to differences in the shape of the bones of the skull. The layer of soft tissue covering the skull is relatively thin and has little effect on head shape except in the more muscular areas of the cheeks and chin. Good hair styling depends on a preliminary study of the shape of the client's head and neck. The choice of style should enhance the appearance of the client by highlighting the pleasing points of head structure, and to some extent decreasing the prominence of any undesirable features. To achieve this the hairdresser must study the shape of the head and neck both from the front and in profile. The shapes are perhaps best seen when the hair is wet and lies close to the head. The following features should be noted.

From the front

Shape of the face

The face is the lower front portion of the head, bounded above by the hair line on the forehead and outlined by the cheeks and chin (see Fig. 10.5). Basic face shapes are usually regarded as round, oval, square, oblong, diamond-shaped, heart-shaped and triangular, though many faces are a mixture of shapes. Face shape depends largely on the length of the face from the hairline to the chin, the width of the face between the zygomatic arches and at forehead level, the shape of the mandible (lower jaw), and the amount of muscle (flesh) in the cheeks.

The widest part of the face is usually determined by the zygomatic arches which join the zygomatic bones to the temporal bones on each side of the head. They are particularly prominent in diamond- and heart-shaped faces. The length and width of the face are approximately equal

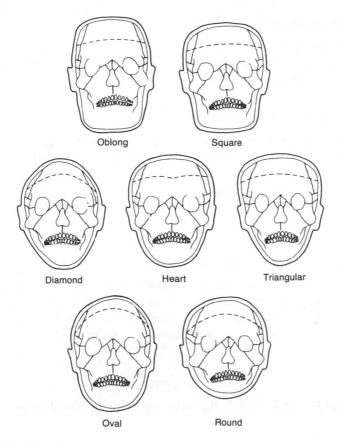

Oblong   Square

Diamond   Heart   Triangular

Oval   Round

Fig. 10.5 Face shapes

in square and round faces, while the length is greater than the width in oval and oblong ones. Square jaws are typical of square and oblong faces, whereas pointed jaws occur in diamond, heart-shaped and triangular faces. The presence of well-formed cheek muscles tends to produce a rounder face, though in older people the cheek muscles often sag and may change the shape of the face to make a squarer jaw line (hence the need for face lifting which raises the muscles of the cheeks).

The **oval shape** is generally considered to be the most desirable and the hair stylist should try to create the illusion of an oval face shape for the client. For example, length in the face may be offset by creating width at the sides using soft waves or curls, width at the temples can be played down by fullness round the chin, and width at the jaw by fullness above chin level.

Dome of the skull

The upper part of the skull may have a high dome or be quite flattened. The height of the head above the forehead hair line must be taken into consideration before styling.

Prominence and size of the ears

Protruding ears are best covered. Clients wearing hearing aids may also ask for the ears to be covered. This cuts down the sound intensity at the hearing aid but may be compensated for by adjusting the volume control. The effect depends partly on the position of the microphone on the aid, which may be forwards facing or situated at the base of the aid behind the ear.

Length and width of the neck

The sterno-mastoid and trapezius muscles contribute to the width of the neck, the platysma at the front of the neck usually consisting only of a very thin sheet of muscle. Neck lengths vary considerably although the basic bone structure always consist of seven vertebrae.

In profile

In profile (see Fig. 10.6) the following features should be observed.

Prominence of the nose

The bones of the nose form only the bridge or upper part of the nose, the tip consisting of cartilage, which is much softer. Emphasis should be taken away from a prominent nose by soft curls at the chin line and avoiding a central parting.

Shape of the chin

The chin may recede or be prominent depending on the shape of the mandible and the amount of muscle in the tip of the chin. In old age, loss of teeth and contraction of the mouth tissues may contribute to the prominence of the chin.

Prominence of the frontal bone in the forehead

Receding foreheads are disguised by full fringes. Narrow foreheads are better with the hair swept back.

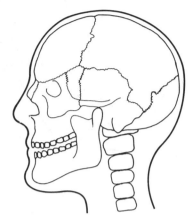 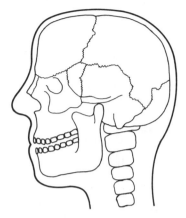

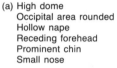

(a) High dome
  Occipital area rounded
  Hollow nape
  Receding forehead
  Prominent chin
  Small nose

(b) Dome of skull flattened
  Occipital area flattened
  No hollow at nape
  Prominent forehead
  Receding chin
  Prominent nose

Fig. 10.6 Features of the head in profile

Shape of the back of the skull

The size of the hollow at the nape depends on the shape of the occipital bone at the back of the skull and the angle at which the neck vertebrae meet the base of the skull.

GROWTH PATTERNS OF HAIR

The angle of inclination of the hair follicles in the skin (see Fig. 10.7), together with the stiffness of the hair, determine the natural lift of hairs, that is how they stand or lie flat to the scalp. The inclination also determines the direction of growth of the hair.

Scalp hairs tend to grow in groups, causing different sections of hair to lie in different directions (see Fig. 10.8). At the crown, for example, the inclination of the follicles causes all the hairs to grow away from one point. Sometimes two such points form a **double crown**. If a natural parting exists, the hair falls easily to each side. At the front margin, the hair may have a tendency to grow forwards, backwards or to one side, possibly forming a **cow lick**. The front hairline may also grow to a point in the centre forehead forming a **widow's peak**. **Whorls** of hair at the nape sometimes make a straight hair line difficult to achieve.

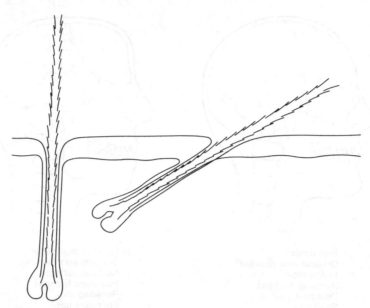

Fig. 10.7 Inclination of the follicle

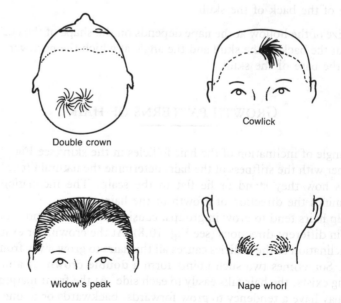

Double crown

Cowlick

Widow's peak

Nape whorl

Fig. 10.8 Growth patterns of hair

The hairdresser must consider the natural lie of the hair when deciding on a suitable style. Growth patterns are most easily seen when the hair is wet. Although disguise of the patterns is possible, forcing the hair against its natural growth can lead to disaster. The style will last longer, keep a better shape and be easier to manage if it follows the natural fall. (The lie of hair is carefully considered by the surgeon when hair transplants are being carried out on bald heads.)

QUANTITY

The quantity of hair or the **hair density** can be measured as the number of hairs per square centimetre and has an average value of around 250 hairs per square centimetre. The quantity of hair usually decreases with age as some follicles cease producing hair. There is in any case a large variation in different people and hair density is best thought of in terms of a thick head of hair, a medium head, and fine or sparse.

Length of hair is also important and a particular style may be impossible if the hair has previously been cut very short. If hair is long, the extra weight of the hair has to be considered when deciding on a style.

TYPE

Types of hair include tightly curled, curly, wavy and straight. Chemical treatment to reduce curl or to increase the curl in straight hair may be necessary according to the style required.

TEXTURE

Texture of hair refers to its diameter or thickness and may be classed as coarse, medium or fine. Coarse hair tends to be strong and wiry. Fine hair is often limp. The diameter depends on the presence of a medulla in the hair, the number of layers of scales in the cuticle, and the thickness and water content of the cortex. Texture also depends on the feel of the hair, whether it is soft and pliable or hard and brittle. This again is affected by the amount of water in the hair shaft and by the roughness of the cuticle scales.

CONDITION

Hair condition was considered in Chapter 9. A hairdresser should always try to discover the reason for poor condition by discussing with the client any past salon treatment, as well as home treatment, and by looking at the client's record card if available. Over-processed hair or very dry hair lacks elasticity and will not produce a good roller set, nor will it blow dry well. Reconditioning (see Chapter 11) may be necessary to ensure good styling and also before any chemical processing can be carried out. Tests to determine hair condition are described later in this chapter.

AGE, PERSONALITY AND LIFESTYLE

Hair styles should be adapted to the needs and personality of the client to ensure a result that gives satisfaction and not embarrassment. Older clients and those of a quiet nature will generally require a subdued hair style; young clients and those with an active social life may prefer something more adventurous; while clients involved in sporting activities may need shorter styles or styles which can be tied back. Consultation with the client is essential.

SELF TESTING

1. What factors may limit the choice of hair style?
2. What is (a) the cranium (b) the mandible?
3. Name the bone which shapes (a) the forehead (b) the back of the head.
4. Which muscles contribute to the width of the neck?
5. How do the contours of the face change with age?
6. What shape of face is considered to be ideal? How does this affect styling?
7. What features of the face are best studied in profile?
8. What is meant by (a) hair density (b) hair texture?
9. On what factors does the diameter of a hair depend?
10. Name four different types of hair growth pattern which influence styling.
11. Why is it advisable to follow natural growth patterns during styling?
12. What effect does lack of elasticity in hair have on styling?

SUITABILITY OF CHEMICAL PROCESSING

Chemical processing should not be carried out without first examining the hair and the skin of the scalp, establishing whether or not previous chemical processing has taken place, and ensuring that the process can be carried out satisfactorily without serious damage to the hair. The client should be asked about previous treatments but the hair should also be examined carefully to determine its condition. Various tests should be carried out before a final decision is made.

Contra-indications to chemical processing

No chemical treatment must be carried out in the following cases.

- If infections or infestations are found on the hair or skin of the scalp.
- If the skin of the scalp is broken by cuts or abrasions. (Very minor defects may be covered by petroleum jelly or barrier cream.) Chemicals entering breaks in the skin can be painful and may sometimes cause allergic reaction.
- If there are chemicals already present on the hair which would react with those to be used during processing, resulting in hair damage. In hairdressing the chemicals involved are said to be **incompatible**.
- If the hair has already been seriously weakened by previous over-processing or other damage.

PROCEDURE BEFORE CHEMICAL PROCESSING

Before any proposed chemical treatment such as permanent waving, bleaching, applying a permanent dye, or removing a permanent colour, the following precautions must be taken. The treatment must not be carried out if there is any doubt about its success.

Examine hair and scalp

Examine the client's hair and scalp skin for signs of infection or infestation, and the skin for cuts and abrasions.

Consult client

Discuss the intended treatment and any previous treatments with the client, especially any home treatment. For an established client, consult the record card.

Incompatibility test

If you are unsure of any home treatment the client may have had, particularly if the hair appears very dark with a dull, flat colour, an incompatibility test is useful. Certain metallic salts used in hair colour restorers and compound henna preparations may react vigorously with the hydrogen peroxide used in perm neutralizers, bleaches and in the application of permanent dyes, causing hair damage and possible breakage of the hair. A small test cutting should be taken from an unnoticeable area of the client's hair and tested in 20 volume hydrogen peroxide. If any vigorous reaction takes place, including the production of bubbles of gas (oxygen) and heat, processing involving the use of hydrogen peroxide should not be carried out. There is no satisfactory method of removing this type of colour and the colour must be allowed to grow out before it is safe to carry out any chemical processing.

Elasticity test

Ensure that the hair is in good enough condition to withstand processing. If the hair is thought to have been over-processed by previous treatment, an elasticity test should be carried out. A single hair or a small group of hairs should be held in two places using the thumb and index finger of both hands some distance apart along the hair shaft and the hair gently pulled with the lower hand. If the hair stretches appreciably without springing back or breaks easily, any further processing should be avoided because the hair shows signs of serious damage to the cortex and further treatment would increase that damage. Hair at different parts of the scalp should be tested.

Porosity test

The hair should also be examined to estimate damage to its surface condition. The rougher the surface the greater the damage to the cuticle and the more porous the hair. Estimating porosity requires some experience because there is no accurate test. A simple porosity test involves taking a strand of several hairs and rubbing them between the fingers, or sliding the fingers along the length of the hair from points to roots against the lie of the cuticle. This will indicate the roughness of the cuticle and give an approximate guide to its porosity. Porous hair absorbs lotions more easily than non-porous hair. Care is required regarding the strength of lotions used and length of processing time when treating porous hair.

Pre-perm lotions

If porosity is uneven along the hair shafts, processing will also be uneven. In the case of perming, pre-perm lotions may be applied to even out porosity. These contain protein hydrolysates (see Chapter 11) or **'fillers'** designed to be applied after the hair has been shampooed and towel dried, and are left on the hair during perming. They cling to the surface of the cuticle and also to damaged bonds in the hair shaft, and help to even out porosity. The manufacturer's instructions should be carefully followed as some perm lotions contain protein hydrolysates and the pre-perm lotion is unnecessary. Similar 'fillers' are available for application before permanent tinting and bleaching.

Further tests before perming

Pre-perm test

A pre-perm test will indicate how much of a previous perm remains in the hair. Perming again over previously permed hair may cause damage and the results could be poor. Ideally the old perm should have grown out before re-perming. The pre-perm test is carried out by examining wet hair after shampooing and towel drying the hair. This removes the effect of setting or blow drying which may have straightened the hair temporarily, and reveals the curl of previous perming.

Test curls

As a precautionary measure a series of test curls may be made if there is uncertainty about the possible success of perming, or if there is doubt about the strength of lotion required, the size of rods to use, or the length of processing time. Using several small sections near the crown, wind, process and neutralize the sections normally, and assess the result. Different rod sizes or lotions of different strengths may be used. The effect on elasticity and tensile strength should be tested after processing. Test curls are particularly useful to test bleached hair or hair where old perm is still present and will indicate the possibility of further damage.

Further test before bleaching

A **test cutting** (sometimes called a **strand test**) may be carried out if you are unsure of the outcome of bleaching due to uncertainty about hair condition or before commencing a full-head bleach. Several small cuttings are taken from different areas of the hair and secured at the root end with adhesive tape. They are treated with the intended bleaching reagents and left until the required lift is achieved. The bleach is then rinsed off and after drying, the hair is tested to note any change in elasticity or tensile strength. The test also acts as an incompatibility test to show the presence of metallic salts on the hair which would cause damage during bleaching, as well as indicating the success of a full-head bleach.

Further tests before using a permanent dye

Skin test

Carry out a skin test 24–48 hours before the proposed application of the dye to avoid the danger of dye dermatitis. A small proportion of people develop an **allergy** to para (permanent) dyes and even a client who has been using para dyes over a long period may suddenly develop a reaction to the dye. It is recommended that a test should be carried out before every proposed application. The mildest symptoms of dye dermatitis are slight itching and redness of the skin round the hair line. More severe symptoms include the swelling of the whole face, the development of papules and general prostration.

The usual skin test is a **Sabouraud–Rousseau test** (also called an allergy test, a patch test, a hypersensitivity test, a predisposition test or an idiosyncrasy test). This is carried out as follows:

- Using surgical spirit on cotton wool, clean a small area of skin either behind the ear close to the hair line, or on the inside of the elbow.
- Mix a small quantity of the same dye and hydrogen peroxide of the same strength as that intended to be used on the client's head and apply a spot about the same size as a 1p coin to the cleaned area of skin and allow to dry.
- Cover the area with collodion, which will leave a clear film over the area.
- Advise the client to leave the patch alone until returning to the salon unless there is irritation and redness. In that case the dye should be washed off and the area treated with calamine lotion.
- Any irritation, however slight, indicates a **positive reaction** to the dye and under no circumstances should the dye be applied to the hair.
- If there is no reaction (sometimes called a **negative reaction** to the skin test) it can be assumed safe to apply the tint.

Test cutting

If there is doubt about the outcome of the dye due to poor hair condition, or there is to be a complete change of colour, a test cutting may be taken from an unnoticeable part of the head and tested with the proposed dye. The cut hair can be kept together by the use of adhesive tape. Suitable development time for the dye is allowed before washing the cutting, then drying and testing it for any change in condition. The suitability of the process can thus be assessed.

Further tests before using a colour reducer (stripper)

Test cutting

A test cutting of the client's hair should be taken from an unnoticeable area and the intended reducer applied. If it is shown that there are no adverse effects to the hair and the reduction process is satisfactory, the colour removal can proceed.

Skin test

If it is intended to use a permanent dye after colour removal, a skin test is also required.

TESTS DURING CHEMICAL PROCESSING

Curl test

During permanent waving, a curl test is used at regular intervals to check the development of the curl and to indicate when the hair is sufficiently processed, so avoiding chemical damage by over-processing. This involves partially unwinding several rods in turn on different parts of the head and gently pushing the hair towards the head. Processing is complete when the hair forms an S-shape of the same size as the diameter of the rod being used.

Strand test

During bleaching or applying a permanent colour, a strand test is required to monitor the development of the bleach or dye, and to decide when processing is complete. This involves removing the bleach or dye from a small section of hair with a damp piece of cotton wool, to show the colour development or to ensure during a retouch that there is no demarkation between the regrowth and the remainder of the hair. Over-processing a bleach may cause serious damage to the hair.

SELF TESTING

1. What is meant by chemicals being 'incompatible'?
2. Describe a test for incompatibility and state its purpose.
3. Explain the circumstances which would make chemical processing of the hair inadvisable.
4. Why is (a) porosity and (b) elasticity important when considering chemical treatment?
5. What is the main ingredient of a pre-perm lotion? What effect does it have on hair?
6. What is a pre-perm test designed to show? Why is it important?
7. Describe how and why you would use test curls before perming.
8. Describe the use of test cuttings before a bleach.
9. Give three alternative names for a skin test. How and when is such a test carried out?
10. What symptoms would show a client had a positive reaction to a para dye?
11. What are the symptoms of dye dermatitis?
12. What tests are carried out during (a) perming (b) bleaching? What is the purpose of these tests?

PART 4

TREATMENTS AND HAIR PROCESSING

CONDITIONING TREATMENTS FOR HAIR AND SCALP

Conditioners may be used to protect hair and maintain good condition during all hairdressing processes, or to improve hair if, for any reason, condition has deteriorated. Many different conditioning agents are available, some designed to be used alone or along with heat or massage treatments, while others are added to products such as shampoos, perm lotions, and permanent dyes.

TYPES OF CONDITIONERS

Conditioners can be grouped into three main types: oil-based, acid, and substantive conditioners.

Oil-based conditioners

Oils are mostly used as surface conditioners applied sparingly to produce a thin oily film on the hair cuticle, replacing the sebum removed during shampooing, or to give a deeper conditioning treatment on very dry hair.
  The oil acts

- as an **emollient** (a substance which softens skin and hair) making the hair both soft and supple
- by **smoothing the hair** so reducing frictional damage when brushing and combing hair and preventing tangling
- by **increasing the reflection** of light so improving gloss or sheen
- as a **moisturizer** by preventing loss of moisture from the hair shaft
- by **controlling wisps**
- by **reducing** the production of **static electricity** on the surface of the hair.

Vegetable oils

Vegetable oils, such as olive oil and almond oil, were formerly frequently used in hot oil conditioning treatments. These treatments have now largely been replaced by the use of oil shampoos followed by cream rinses containing cetrimide. Castor oil and almond oil are occasionally used in dressing creams and control creams.

Mineral oils

Mineral oils, such as paraffin jelly and liquid paraffin, are the usual ingredients of dressing creams, control creams, brilliantines, and hair sprays designed to control hair and add shine.

Lanolin

Lanolin (wool fat similar to sebum) and synthetic products made to resemble sebum are added as conditioners to cream shampoos, cream rinses, hair dyes, lacquers and conditioning creams. Conditioning creams take the form of oil-in-water emulsions, the oils being left on the hair when the water evaporates. Heat, by use of hot towels or a steamer, is often used to ensure good penetration of conditioning cream or oils between the cuticle scales. (The use of lanolin itself is now less popular as it is known to cause allergy in some people. Its presence in a hair preparation must be stated on the label.)

Silicone oils

Silicone oils or silicone fluids, such as dimethyl silicone (dimethicone), are increasingly used as conditioners in shampoos, setting lotions, perm lotions, lacquers and cream rinses. They are also used in restructurants to repair split ends by temporarily 'glueing' the ends together. Silicone oils are heat resistant so are particularly suitable in setting lotions used during blow drying, leaving a very fine, soft, water-resistant film which is also antistatic. Some silicones are in the form of polymers, that is a large number of silicone molecules combined together to form a single molecule of polymer ('poly' means many). Silicone polymers are sometimes referred to as **protective polymer conditioners**.

Acid conditioners

Weak acids can act as both surface and penetrating conditioners. Traditionally, weak organic acids such as acetic acid (vinegar), citric acid (in lemon juice) and tartaric acid were used as neutralizing rinses after using soap shampoos which were always alkaline, and to remove any deposits of lime soap if the water was hard. In salons soap shampoos have now been replaced by non-alkaline soapless detergents and this use for acid conditioners no longer exists. In modern hairdressing weak organic acids have other uses.

Uses of acids as conditioners

* Citric acid is an ingredient of **pH balanced soapless shampoos** giving a pH of about 6 which ensures that the hair is left in its normally slightly acid state after shampooing. Most modern shampoos are acidic.
* Organic acids to give a pH of about 4 are used as rinses or **pH restorers** to chemically neutralize any alkali left on the hair after perming, tinting and bleaching. Ascorbic acid (vitamin C) is often preferred for this purpose as it is also an **anti-oxidant** and helps to stop the action of hydrogen peroxide after processing is completed. Acids also help to stop the loss of soluble protein material from the hair produced by chemical damage during perming and bleaching.

Substantive conditioners

Hair keratin is made up of long chains of amino acids called polypeptide chains. Along the chains spare amino groups (positively charged) and spare acid groups (negatively charged) form side branches. When an acid group lies opposite to an amino group in an adjacent chain a salt linkage is formed, but many of the groups are unattached or free (see Fig. 11.1). Substantive conditioners have an electrical charge and so are attracted electrostatically to the free amino groups or the free acid groups in the hair. They become attached to keratin either on the cuticle or inside the hair shaft and some of the conditioner remains attached even after the hair has been rinsed and dried. There are actually more free acid groups (negatively charged groups) than free amino groups in keratin, so many substantive conditioners carry a positive charge. (Remember that opposite electrical charges attract each other and like charges repel each other.) Substantive conditioners include cationic detergents, plastic resins such as polyvinyl pyrrolidone, and protein hydrolysates.

Cationic detergents

Cationic detergents include quaternary ammonium compounds, such as cetrimide (**cetyl trimethyl ammonium bromide**), which carry a positive

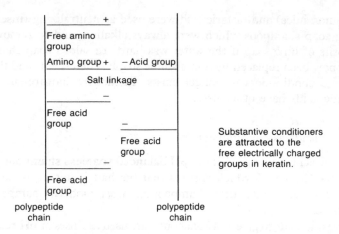

Fig. 11.1 Free charged groups in keratin

electrical charge so will cling to the negatively charged acid groups in the hair.

Cetrimide

- Prevents the production of static electrical charges on hair, making it easier to comb with less tangling.
- acts as an emollient making the hair softer (cetrimide is also used in laundry work as a fabric softener).
- acts as a humectant by attracting water to the hair shaft.
- is used in conditioning rinses (cream rinses) after shampooing. The number of acid groups in hair increases when the hair is chemically damaged, so more cetrimide is taken up by damaged hair. (Most shampoos have a negative charge so that it is important to wash out the shampoo before using the rinse. The opposite charge on the shampoo would destroy the effect of the conditioner.)
- is used as a conditioner added to setting lotions, lacquers, perm lotions, and as an after-treatment conditioner for perms, bleaches and tints.

Polyvinyl pyrrolidone

Polyvinyl pyrrolidone (PVP), a plastic resin, is added to shampoos and cold wave lotions and acts as a humectant or water-attracting agent which helps to add extra water to the hair shaft, making the hair feel softer.

Protein hydrolysates

Protein hydrolysates contain amino acid molecules, either singly or in short chains, which are attracted electrostatically to electrically charged groups inside the hair and form bonds similar to the salt linkages in keratin. Protein hydrolysates are made by breaking down waste protein materials such as horse hair, feathers, collagen from hides, or from vegetable proteins such as soya beans, by a process called hydrolysis. (This process involves the breakdown of a substance with the addition of the elements of water to the new substances formed.)

Protein hydrolysates are used

- as conditioning '**fillers**' before perming, bleaching or permanent colouring. Protein hydrolysates may contain both free acids groups or free amino groups which will be attracted to the free groups of the hair. They cling to damaged bonds in the hair shaft, even out porosity by filling in spaces in the hair structure, and prevent the uneven uptake of chemicals during processing so avoiding patchy results. They also help to prevent the loss of protein material damaged during processing which would otherwise be washed out of the hair.
- as conditioners in some perm lotions to work in the same way as 'fillers'.
- in shampoos for use on damaged hair.
- in setting lotions to make the hair smoother and more lustrous.

Other conditioners

Alkaline substances such as borax and ammonium hydroxide are sometimes used as rinses to help to remove excess grease in cases of seborrhoea. Some **rehabilitating rinses** mostly for home use include various **herbs** including camomile, to give slight colour and highlights to blonde hair; **henna** may be used as conditioner on dark hair; **beer** rinses and **egg** rinses give 'body' and shine.

RESTRUCTURANTS

A restructurant is a product designed to improve the structure of hair, particularly the internal structure.

There are several types:

- **Cationic detergents** were among the earliest restructurants. They have a positive charge and are attracted to negatively charged acid groups in the hair, e.g. hydroxymethyl imidazolinethione in an acid solution.

- **Protein hydrolysates** are substantive to hair and form bonds similar to the salt linkages of the hair. They may be linked chemically with quaternary ammonium compounds to increase the uptake of amino acids into the hair.
- Some recent restructurants are based on the development of **plastic polymers** such as poly methylmethacrylate inside the hair shaft.
- **Silicone based** restructurants are used to repair split ends by temporarily 'glueing' the ends together.

USES OF CONDITIONERS

Preventing loss of condition due to chemical processing

Before chemical processing

Use pre-perm 'fillers' containing protein hydrolysates to counteract varying porosity along the hair shafts and lessen damage during processing.

Similarly use 'fillers' before applying permanent dyes and before bleaching.

After chemical processing

Use acid anti-oxidant rinses immediately after perming, bleaching or permanent dyeing. They contain mild reducing agents such as ascorbic acid with additional citric acid to give a pH of 4. They halt the oxidation process, neutralize the alkali left on the hair after processing, and prevent loss of soluble protein material produced by chemical damage.

For later follow-up treatment use protein shampoos and cetrimide cream rinses.

Improving hair in poor condition

Poor surface condition

Poor surface condition is improved by:

- **acids** of pH 6 to reduce swelling of the hair shaft and smooth the cuticle scales
- **oils** and conditioning creams to improve shine and prevent loss of moisture from the hair
- **restructurants** and protein hydrolysate fillers to treat damaged cuticles and reduce porosity.

Poor internal condition

Poor internal condition due to damage by perming or bleaching is improved by:

- **protein shampoos**
- **substantive conditioners** (cream rinses containing cetrimide).

Treating specific conditions

Hair conditions

- **Fragilitas crinium** (split ends): cut where possible or treat with substantive conditioners or restructurants.
- **Damaged cuticle**: use restructurants or protein hydrolysates.
- **Dry over-processed hair**: use conditioning creams, moisturizers or cetrimide cream rinses.
- **Trichorrhexis nodosa**: use restucturants or protein hydrolysates.

Scalp conditions

- **Pityriasis capitis** (simple dandruff): use oily conditioners or conditioning creams to counteract dryness. Use anti-dandruff shampoos containing zinc pyrithione to reduce scaling.
- **Seborrhoea** (excessive oiliness): apply astringent or spirit lotions to the skin of the scalp. Use shampoos designed for greasy hair containing increased amounts of detergent, and alkaline rinses.

SELF TESTING

1. In what ways are oils useful as conditioners?
2. What is meant by (a) an emollient (b) a moisturizer (c) a humectant?
3. What type of oil is usually used in dressing or control creams?
4. What is lanolin? In what products is it used? What is the disadvantage of using lanolin?
5. What are the main uses of silicone oils?
6. What is meant by a pH balanced shampoo?
7. Name three substantive conditioners. What does substantive mean?
8. What is the main use of cetrimide?
9. Why must a soapless shampoo be rinsed out of the hair before applying a cetrimide rinse?

10. What is a protein hydrolysate? What type of conditioners contain protein hydrolysates?
11. What is the purpose of an alkaline rinse?
12. What type of conditioner is used (a) before chemical treatments (b) after chemical treatments?
13. What type of conditioner is used to treat (a) fragilitas crinium (b) trichorrexis nodosa?
14. What is pityriasis capitis? How should it be treated in a salon?

HEAT TREATMENTS

Heat treatments increase the blood supply to the scalp by causing the small blood vessels (capillaries) in the dermis to dilate, that is to become wider. This causes redness of the skin or **erythema**. The extra blood flow, known as **hyperaemia**, brings more nutrients (glucose and amino acids) and oxygen to the scalp so encouraging hair growth, and also makes the sebaceous glands more active. Heat treatments used with conditioning agents, such as conditioning creams or vegetable oils, will enable the oils to penetrate between the cuticle scales as heat causes swelling of the hair shaft and lifts the scales. For hot oil treatment a vegetable oil such as olive oil is heated to 55°C and brushed on to the hair. Heat may be applied by use of hot towels, or a steamer or an infra-red heater, and may be used in conjunction with massage of the scalp before and/or after heating.

Note

- Oil treatments must not be given immediately before chemical processing such as perming, bleaching, or tinting because the oil could create a barrier which prevents lotions entering the hairshaft.

Hot towels

Hot towels produce a moist heat and are prepared by soaking the towel in water at 60°C, then wringing out well before wrapping tightly round the client's head. A series of hot towels is required as they must be replaced as soon as they cool.

Steamers

Steamers consist basically of an electric kettle with a hood to direct the steam over the client's head (see Fig. 11.2) so producing a moist heat

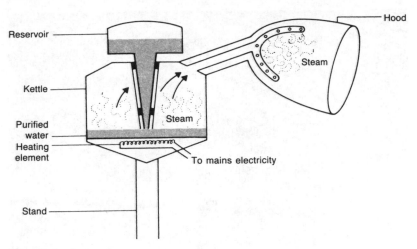

Fig. 11.2 A steamer

treatment. Purified water (distilled or de-ionized) should be used in the steamer to prevent loss of efficiency by 'scale' deposits from hard water which may accumulate in the kettle or block the steam outlets.

Infra-red lamps

Infra-red lamps, sometimes called **accelerators**, produce a dry heat as opposed to the moist heat of a steamer. Hand models are available containing a 275 watt infra-red lamp. Stand models have a cluster of three or five lamps mounted on flexible arms which can be positioned as desired (see Fig. 11.3). In other models less powerful lamps are arranged in groups along movable arms. More recently **roller balls** have been introduced: using a motor to keep the infra-red lamps moving and avoiding the development of 'hot spots'. Infra-red lamps are similar to the filament lamps used for lighting, but the filament operates at a lower temperature. They have a silvered internal reflector to reflect the invisible heat rays downwards through a red glass cover which cuts out some of the light rays. Heat travels from the lamp by radiation in straight lines.

Safety notes

- Care should be taken in positioning infra-red lamps as they may cause burns if too close to the client and eye damage if the rays are directed on to the eyes.
- The lamps themselves become very hot and should not be touched during or immediately after use.

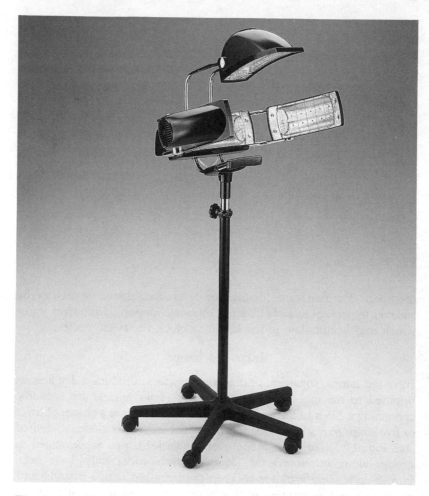

Fig. 11.3 Infra-red heater

MASSAGE

Massage of the scalp is normally carried out by hand. Mechanical massage using a vibro massage machine is possible but is now rarely practised. During massage the scalp is moved over the bones of the skull, the movement being possible due to the very loose connection between the scalp and the bone (see the structure of the scalp in Chapter 7 including Fig. 7.1).

Contra-indications to use of massage

Massage should not be carried out in the following cases.

- If there are cuts and abrasions on the scalp.
- When any infections or infestations are present on the scalp or hair.
- On inflamed skin.
- Where there are septic conditions, e.g. boils.
- If the client has a heart condition or problems with blood circulation.
- If the hair is very greasy.
- Prior to perming, bleaching, or tinting the hair.

Effect of massage

- The main effect of massage is to produce hyperaemia or increased blood flow to the scalp. This aids the supply of nutrients to the hair follicles and encourages hair growth. At the same time waste products are removed more quickly from the area.
- The sebaceous glands are stimulated to produce more sebum so particularly benefiting clients with dry hair.
- Clients usually find massage to be relaxing, and tension is reduced.

Hand massage

Hand massage should be carried out smoothly and rhythmically without any jerkiness. The hairdresser's nails should be kept short and smooth to prevent scratching the scalp or catching in the hair. The hands and wrists should always be flexible and never held stiffly. A complete massage normally takes no more than 15 minutes. A shorter massage may be more appropriate for older clients or those new to the treatment.

There are five hand massage movements, though in hairdressing effleurage, petrissage and frictions are most commonly used.

Effleurage

Effleurage is a slow stroking movement involving a firm yet light pressure with the palms of the hands or the pads of the fingertips starting at the forehead and finishing at the nape or top of the shoulder in one continuous movement. It is used at the beginning and end of treatment because it has a soothing and relaxing effect.

Petrissage

Petrissage is the main movement for scalp massage and involves circular motions with the fingers spread out in a claw-like position with one hand on each side of the scalp. The right hand moves in a clockwise direction and the left hand anti-clockwise. The aim is to move the scalp over the skull in a kneading action. The fingertips should be firmly pressed to the scalp so that there is no movement of the fingers over the scalp until they glide to repeat the treatment on another area.

Frictions

Frictions involve small circular movements with pressure applied to move the scalp over the skull with the fingertips and thumbs rather than to just rub the skin. The kneading movements are quicker than in petrissage but the fingers are still rotated in opposite directions for each hand. Frictions are used on the scalp when shampooing or applying lotions.

Vibrations

Vibrations involve a shaking or trembling movement with the finger pads placed firmly against the skin. Light vibrations are soothing and heavier ones more stimulating. As an aid to this type of massage an electrical vibrator may be strapped to the back of the hand while the fingertips rest on the scalp and will produce either weak or strong vibrations.

Tapotement

Tapotement is a tapping or patting movement rarely used on the scalp.

Vibro massage

A vibro massage machine is electrically operated and for scalp massage is fitted with a rubber pronged or spiked applicator which moves with a to-and-fro or vibratory action. This gives a type of massage similar to frictions in hand massage. The prongs should be held lightly but firmly against the skin without any added pressure, and the applicator lifted occasionally to avoid tangling the hair. The machine may be used in small circular movements to cover the surface of the scalp or in straight lines from the front hair line to the nape. The method is now rarely used in salons.

HIGH FREQUENCY TREATMENTS

High frequency is a means of scalp treatment using an oscillating or alternating electric current. The treatment produces hyperaemia, that is increased blood flow to the scalp, and so brings more nutrients and oxygen to the follicles encouraging hair growth. Used frequently over a period of time it may benefit cases of hair loss (alopecia).

What is a high frequency current?

Mains electricity is said to be an alternating current because the flow of electrons which creates the current (see Chapter 5 for details of electrons and mains electricity) changes direction or alternates 100 times every second, that is in every second it flows 50 times in one direction and 50 in the other. This is called a frequency or frequence of 50 cycles per second or 50 hertz (50 Hz) and is a low frequency current. The high frequency machine increases this frequency to 500 000 hertz. Mains voltage of 240 volts is also increased to around 2000 volts but the current size (amps) is very small. The rapid alternation of current in the skin creates heat causing dilation of the blood vessels in the dermis.

High frequency machine

The high frequency machine (see **Fig. 11.4**) has three parts:

- the mains power supply
- a control box containing an oscillatory circuit which changes the current to one of high voltage and high frequency but of very low strength or amperage which will not produce an electric shock when applied to the client's scalp; the control box also has an on/off switch and an intensity control to vary the strength of current
- a circuit from the control box to apply the high frequency current either directly to the scalp through a glass electrode inserted in an insulating plastic holder, or indirectly through a metal electrode or saturator held by the client.

Contra-indications to high frequency treatment

High frequency treatment must not be carried out in the following cases.

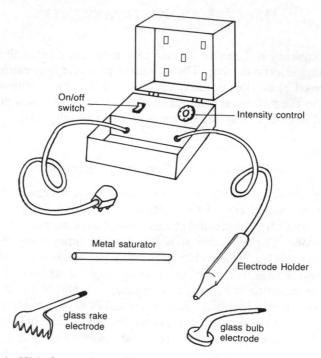

Fig. 11.4 High frequency machine

- Heart conditions or high blood pressure.
- Infections or infestations of the scalp or hair.
- Cuts, abrasions or inflammation on the scalp.
- Excessively greasy hair because treatment increases sebum production.
- Headaches, migraine or epilepsy.
- Nervousness or fear of electric currents.
- Pregnancy.

Precautions is use of high frequency treatment

- Before use check the high frequency equipment for damaged flexes, faulty plugs or cracked electrodes.
- Ask the client to remove jewellery including earrings. Check that jewellery from your own hands and wrists has been removed.
- Avoid working near metal objects or in wet areas.
- High frequency treatment should only be carried out on dry hair.
- Do not use spirit lotions on the hair: they are flammable and sparking could ignite them.
- Glass electrodes should be pushed rather than pulled through the hair. Pulling may dislodge the electrode from the holder.

Direct method of high frequency treatment

This method involves applying the high frequency current directly to the scalp by means of a glass electrode. The glass electrode is hollow and is a partial vacuum to allow the current or stream of electrons to flow through. The electrode should be placed in the holder or handle before switching on the current.

Starting with a low current the operator should keep in finger contact with the electrode until the electrode is safely in contact with the client's scalp. This prevents sparking between the electrode and scalp which may be uncomfortable and even frightening for the client. Alternatively the electrode should be placed in contact with the scalp before switching on the current and with the current control at zero. The current may be increased gradually during treatment but should never be uncomfortable for the client.

Avoid lifting the electrode away from the scalp during treatment or again sparking may occur as the current jumps across the air gap. Similarly at the end of treatment the current should be returned to zero and only then switched off before removing the electrode from the scalp, or the operator must again keep in finger contact with the electrode before removing it from the scalp and switching off.

There are two types of glass electrode: a flat round bulb and a glass rake.

Flat round bulb

A flat round bulb is drawn with a circular movement over patches of bare skin in cases of alopecia areata. This increases the blood flow to the area and encourages new hair growth but to be effective a series of treatments is required.

Glass rake

A glass rake is used on a normal scalp or on areas where the hair is thinning. The rake is pushed through the hair from the hair line to the crown.

Indirect method of high frequency treatment

This method involves the use of a metal bar electrode or **saturator**. The client holds the metal bar in one hand and the insulated handle in the other hand while the operator massages the client's scalp. The current passes from the bar through the client's body and to earth through the operator's hands. To avoid sparking, the current should not be switched either on or off unless the operator's hand is in contact with the scalp.

Cleaning the electrodes

After use on a client, the electrodes should be disinfected by use of an alcohol wipe. They should be stored in a clean place or preferably in an ultra-violet cabinet ready for re-use.

SELF TESTING

1. What is meant by (a) hyperaemia (b) erythema?
2. What type of oil is used in a hot oil treatment? At what temperature is the oil applied?
3. State three methods by which heat can be applied to the scalp.
4. Why should hot oil treatment never be given immediately before a perm or bleach?
5. Why should purified water be used in a steamer?
6. What precautions should be taken when using infra-red lamps?
7. What effect does massage have on the scalp?
8. Name five movements used in hand massage. Which three are most commonly used on the scalp?
9. Which massage movement is most soothing? When and how is it carried out?
10. Which types of massage involve a kneading action? How are the movements carried out?
11. What type of applicator is used directly on the scalp in vibro massage? What type of massage does it provide? How is the massage carried out?
12. What are the contra-indications to (a) massage (b) high frequency treatment?
13. What is the effect of high frequency treatment?
14. What is alopecia areata? Which type of glass electrode is used in its treatment?
15. How would you prevent 'sparking' happening during high frequency treatment?
16. Describe the indirect method of high frequency treatment.

12

SHAMPOOING HAIR

The purpose of shampooing is to cleanse the hair and scalp by removal of dust, dirt, grease (mainly sebum), dead skin scales and hairdressing preparations such as dressing creams or lacquer. The shampoo should leave the hair in the best possible condition in preparation for any further hairdressing treatments such as perming, blow waving or cutting. Deposits left on the hair may block perms or leave the hair too greasy for successful blow drying. The hair and scalp should be carefully examined before shampooing to assess condition. If signs of serious infectious disease, infestation or injury are revealed, neither shampooing nor any other treatment can be carried out.

SUBSTANCES USED TO CLEAN HAIR

Substances used to clean hair include solvents, dry absorbent powders, and detergents.

Solvents

Solvents, which work by dissolving grease, have very limited use for cleaning hair except in the cleaning of wigs and postiche. Tetrachloroethane is now used for this purpose. Cleaning should take place in a well-ventilated room away from the clients. Gloves should be worn because the solvent is very degreasing to the skin. Dry cleaning solvents are never used on a client's head.

Dry absorbent powders

Dry powder shampoos contain absorbent powders such as talc, starch, fuller's earth and French chalk, together with an alkali, usually borax or sodium carbonate (washing soda). They are used only in cases where it is impossible to apply a detergent shampoo and water, perhaps because the person is bedfast or for some reason is unable to be shampooed at a salon basin.

A typical formulation is:

> Absorbent powder 80–85 per cent
> Alkali (powder) 15–20 per cent
> Perfume as required

The mixture is sprinkled over the hair section by section in 2 cm partings, and is applied to the hair itself rather than to the scalp. The powder is left for 10–15 minutes to absorb the grease from the hair and is then brushed out systematically, the brush being wiped frequently on a clean towel to remove the dirt and powder. The method is not very satisfactory as it is difficult to remove all traces of powder, and this leaves the hair dull. Since brushing stimulates the activity of the sebaceous glands, hair tends to become greasy quickly after this type of shampoo.

Detergents

Detergents (also called surface active agents or surfactants) include both soaps and soapless (non-soap) detergents and are used in conjunction with water. The detergents used for shampoos are designed to produce a good lather. This helps to keep a concentrated solution of shampoo in close contact with the hair and scalp, enabling the detergent to move easily over the surfaces and so reducing frictional damage to the hair. The lather also acts as a guide to the amount of detergent required. Using more shampoo than is necessary is wasteful. The structure of detergents and their action in cleaning hair will be considered fully later in the chapter. About 20 litres of water at 40°C (just above body temperature) are required while carrying out each shampoo and a good supply of both hot and cold water is therefore essential.

SALON WATER SUPPLY

Cold water enters the salon by a service pipe from an underground mains supply and the water then must be heated as required. The pressure of mains water carries cold water to a tank placed high in the building, the level of water in the tank being controlled by a ball valve (see Fig. 12.1). Cold water from the tank then supplies the hot water tank, toilets and shampoo basins. Some appliances may be connected directly to the

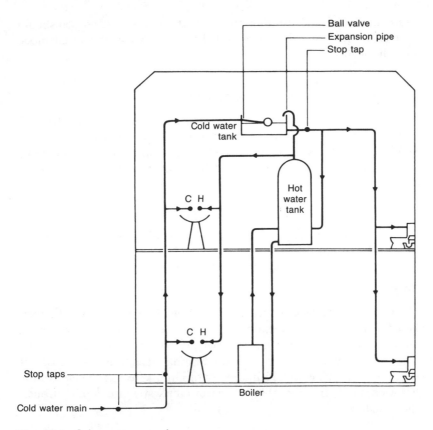

Fig. 12.1 Salon water supply

cold water mains, e.g. instantaneous water heaters. Drinking water should be taken only from taps connected directly to the mains supply, as water which has passed through the cold tank may be contaminated by dust, etc.

Stop taps and meters

Stop taps enable the water supply to be cut off for repairs, for the replacement of tap washers if taps drip, or if there are bursts in the water pipes. The main stop tap is close to the entry point of the supply from outside; a second is on the outlet from the cold water tank. Water for salons is now often metered so that payment is made according to the amount of water used. The meter is installed near the inlet to the building before the main stop tap. To cut costs, both for water itself and its heating, continuously running the water throughout a shampoo should be avoided; the water should be turned off while massaging the shampoo into the scalp.

Safety notes

- Make sure you know the position of stop taps and can turn them off in an emergency: they are sometimes stiff from lack of use.
- If the building is to be left unoccupied for some time, e.g. a holiday period, turn them off to prevent flooding in case of burst pipes.

Hot water supply

There are various methods of heating water for salon use and it is essential to have a constantly available supply.

Boiler

Hot water may be supplied from a boiler heated by oil, gas, or solid fuel. Hot water rises by convection from the boiler to the top of a storage tank or cylinder from which it is drawn off to the basins (see Fig. 12.1). The boiler may form part of a central heating system, in which case hot water for the taps is heated indirectly through a heat exchanger in the hot water tank, and is kept separate from the water circulating through the radiators.

Immersion heater

Water may be heated directly in the storage tank by an immersion heater. Heating often takes place at night using cheap off-peak electricity, but in salons with small tanks heating may be required during the day as well. The heating element is enclosed in a metal sheath and may be inserted vertically from the top of the tank (see Fig. 12.2) or horizontally at either the top or bottom. Fitting an immersion heater at the top results in a quick accumulation of hot water at the top of the tank while the bottom remains cold. Hot water rises and since water is a poor conductor of heat no heat passes down the tank. A horizontal heater fitted at the bottom of the tank results in the gradual heating of the whole tank, since the water is constantly circulating by convection. Two-element heaters are available. These are fitted vertically and have a long element to heat the bulk of the water at night using off-peak electricity and a short element to keep the top part of the cylinder hot during the day. The temperature of the water in the hot tank is usually controlled at about 60°C by an adjustable thermostat.

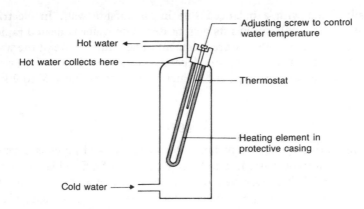

Adjusting screw to control
water temperature

Hot water ←

Hot water collects here

Thermostat

Heating element in
protective casing

Cold water →

Fig. 12.2 Immersion heater

Instantaneous water heater

Instantaneous water heaters are connected to the cold water supply and
the water is heated only as required. The temperature of the water is
usually controlled by a thermostat. They are economical to run and are
particularly suitable for the small salon. Both gas and electrically heated
models are available. In gas heaters (see Fig. 12.3), a small pilot light
constantly burning inside the heater lights the main jet as soon as the
water begins to flow. Single point heaters may be fitted for each basin
or a larger multipoint heater may supply several basins. The heaters are

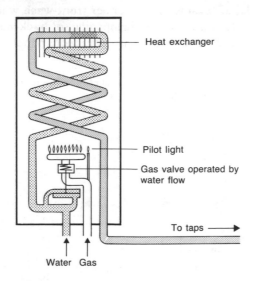

Heat exchanger

Pilot light

Gas valve operated by
water flow

To taps →

Water Gas

Fig. 12.3 Instantaneous water heater

usually fitted with a balanced flue in an outside wall. In electrical installations each basin has its own heater. The water is heated rapidly as it passes over a high powered element. The temperature of the water is thermostatically regulated and depends on the rate of flow of the water and the loading of the appliance which may vary from 3 kW to 9 kW.

Lagging

The insulation or lagging of hot water cylinders and pipes is essential if heat is not to be wasted. The lagging consists of a fitted jacket of any material which is a poor conductor of heat (see Fig. 12.4). Some hot water cylinders have a permanent outer insulating coat of a hard plastic material.

Cold water pipes on cold outer walls and tanks in unheated roof space also require lagging as a protection from frost damage. When water freezes it increases in volume by about one-tenth. This expansion causes great pressure which may burst pipes or damage appliances. Glass-fibre, foam rubber or wool felting are suitable insulating materials.

SHAMPOO BASINS

Shampoo basins are usually made of glazed stoneware or vitreous china which is easily kept clean using a non-abrasive cleaner. Cracked or chipped basins will harbour germs and collect grease and dirt so should always be replaced. Basins may be either **front-wash** where the client lowers the head forwards during shampooing, or **back-wash** where the client lies backwards. Back-wash basins are more popular because they

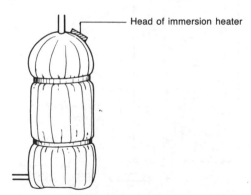

Head of immersion heater

Fig. 12.4   Lagging jacket for hot water cylinder

reduce the possibility of chemicals entering the client's eyes and interfere less with the client's make-up. For client comfort a **chair** of suitable height is essential. Where several basins are connected to the same supply pipe, turning the tap in one basin may affect the flow in an adjacent basin. This is dangerous and may lead to scalding. The problem is overcome if the pipes to the basins have a smaller diameter than that of the main supply pipe.

Features of salon basins

- A **filter** over the opening to the waste pipe to collect hair and prevent it from blocking the drain.
- A **trap** in the waste pipe under the basin with a water seal which prevents unpleasant odours and airborne bacteria entering the salon from the drains. An **S-trap** is shown in Fig. 12.5 and a **bottle trap** in Fig. 12.6. The latter is often preferred as it is more easily cleaned.

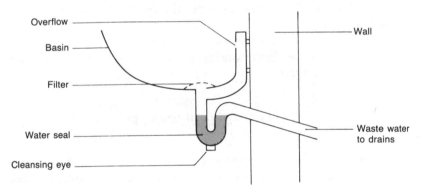

Fig. 12.5 Basin with S-trap

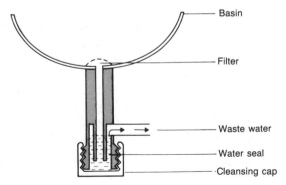

Fig. 12.6 Basin with bottle trap

The cleaning eye or cap can be removed to extract accumulations of solid waste.

- **Mixer taps** which enable the temperature of the water to be easily adjusted. These are sometimes controlled by a valve so that when the desired mix of hot and cold water has been achieved, the tap can be turned on and off without altering the mix.
- A **spray fitting** to the mixer tap to assist shampooing. If salon water is hard, the holes in the spray may gradually become blocked by scale so reducing the efficiency of the spray. The spray head may be removed for cleaning and descaling.

Safety notes

- To prevent scalds when using mixer taps, turn on the cold water first, then add hot water to adjust to the correct temperature.
- Test the temperature of the water on the back of your own hand before using on the client.
- Sensitivity to hot water varies so ask the client if the temperature is satisfactory.
- Treat scalds by running cold water over the area for about 5 minutes.
- Avoid shock to the client by using water which is neither too hot nor too cold for comfort.

HARDNESS OF WATER

Many substances will dissolve in water so that in nature water is rarely pure. A substance which dissolves in water is said to be **soluble** in the water. If it will not dissolve it is **insoluble**. The substance dissolving is called the **solute** and the water the **solvent**. Together they form a **solution**.

Tap water often contains substances which have dissolved in rainwater as it runs through the ground on its way to a reservoir. For example in limestone or chalky areas the water may contain calcium or magnesium salts, but in areas of granite rock the water is relatively free from dissolved salts. Water from the reservoir is purified and made fit for drinking before entering the water mains but still may contain dissolved salts which present no hazard to health. Some of these dissolved salts may be a nuisance to the hairdresser, however, if they may make the water 'hard'.

- **Soft water** contains few dissolved salts and forms an immediate lather with soap.

- **Hard water** contains dissolved salts which form an insoluble scum or curd with soap before forming a lather. Hardness can be temporary or permanent.

Temporary hardness

This type of hardness is due to calcium bicarbonate or magnesium bicarbonate dissolved in water. These salts are formed when rainwater, made acid by dissolving carbon dioxide from the air, reacts with limestone or chalk as it runs through the ground.

Calcium carbonate + carbon dioxide + water → calcium bicarbonate
(insoluble chalk $\underbrace{\qquad\qquad\qquad}$ (soluble in water)
or limestone)   carbonic acid

Temporary hardness can be removed by boiling the water, when the above reaction is reversed and the calcium bicarbonate is decomposed or split up as follows:

Calcium bicarbonate → calcium carbonate + carbon dioxide + water
(insoluble scale)

Calcium carbonate is insoluble and is deposited as a **fur** or **scale**. This deposit takes place in kettles, water pipes, and boilers in hard water areas. Scale also collects in the holes of the spray fittings of shampoo basins and cuts the flow of water. Unless **purified water** is used in steamers, scale may collect in the same way as in a kettle and can also block the steam outlets.

Permanent hardness

This type of hardness is caused by calcium sulphate or magnesium sulphate which is dissolved from the ground by rainwater. Permanent hardness cannot be removed by boiling, but is removed along with temporary hardness using chemical means.

Disadvantages of hard water

Scum

A scum or curd of calcium soap (lime soap) is formed when soap is used in hard water. This wastes soap, as no lather is formed until all the calcium and magnesium salts have reacted with the soap.

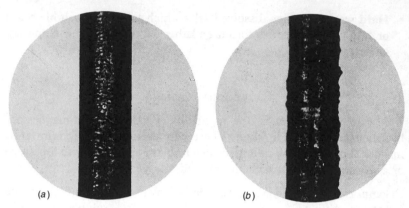

Fig. 12.7(a) Hair washed with soap in soft water **(b)** Hair washed with soap in hard water

Calcium sulphate + sodium stearate → sodium sulphate + calcium stearate
(permanent hardness)   (soap)   (soluble)   (insoluble scum)

No scum is formed if soapless detergents are used instead of soap. Soapless detergent shampoos are thus more satisfactory for use in hard water areas, and most modern shampoos are of this type. The use of soap shampoos in hard water results in a sticky deposit of scum on the hair (see Fig. 12.7) and round the shampoo basin.

Fur

Temporary hardness produces fur or scale deposits in kettles, steamers, pipes and boilers. The circulation of water through central heating pipes may be impeded or stopped if the pipes become blocked. The scale is costly to remove and is damaging to equipment, besides making it less efficient.

Advantages or hard water

The disadvantages of hard water far exceed the slight advantage of a more pleasing taste, and a minor addition of calcium to the diet.

Methods of softening water

If water is hard, it usually contains salts causing both temporary and permanent hardness, though not necessarily in the same proportions. Both types of hardness can be removed by the following methods.

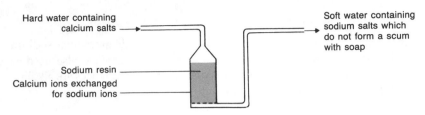

Fig. 12.8 Water softener

Ion exchange

The ion exchange process (Permutit process) is the most satisfactory method for a salon, as the whole supply (except that intended for drinking water) is softened by passing it through a water softener (see Fig. 12.8). This contains sodium ion-exchange resin which exchanges its sodium ions for the calcium ions in the hard water.

sodium resin +calcium sulphate→ calcium resin +sodium sulphate
(water softener)   (in hard water)   (left in the   (dissolved in the
water softener)   softened water)

The water leaving the softener is not chemically pure as it contains dissolved sodium salts, but these do not form a scum with soap so the water is soft. The sodium resin in the water softener is gradually used up, and is replaced by calcium resin which will not soften water. However, the sodium resin may be reformed or regenerated by passing a strong solution of sodium chloride (common salt) through the water softener. This regeneration takes place automatically in modern water softeners.

calcium resin + sodium chloride → sodium resin + calcium chloride
(salt)   (regenerated)   (in water run
to waste)

Water softeners used to contain a natural resin known as zeolite.

Sequestering agent

Sodium hexametaphosphate, which is marketed under the trademark of 'Calogen', is a sequestering agent (to sequester means to separate) and combines with calcium and magnesium ions, preventing the reaction between the soap and hard water, so that no scum is formed. Calgon is often added to shampoo and washing powders as a water softener. It is also used as a rinse after a soap shampoo to remove lime soap from the hair.

Other water softeners

Other water softeners used in laundry work include ammonia, sodium carbonate (washing soda) and borax. Sodium carbonate is also used as a water softener in the form of bath salts. All these substances are alkaline and are not suitable for salon use.

PURIFIED WATER

Chemically pure water is required in the salon for use in the steamer and to dilute chemicals such as hydrogen peroxide. Purified water may be obtained from tap water by either distillation or de-ionization.

Distillation

Distillation is a physical change involving the boiling of impure water to form steam, condensing the steam and collecting the pure water in a clean vessel. The apparatus used is shown in Fig. 12.9. Any impurities are left behind in the flask.

De-ionization

De-ionization involves a chemical process similar to that of ion exchange water softening, but two columns of ion exchange resins are required (see Fig. 12.10a). De-ionized water is more often used than distilled water, as it is easier and cheaper to prepare. The portable de-ionizer shown in Fig. 12.10b contains a replaceable cartridge of resins and gives an immediate supply of de-ionized water when connected to a cold water tap.

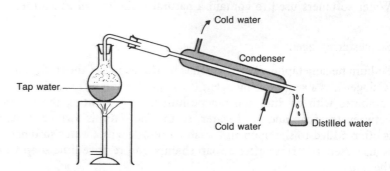

Fig. 12.9   Distillation

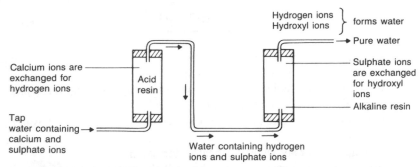

Fig. 12.10(a)   De-ionization of water

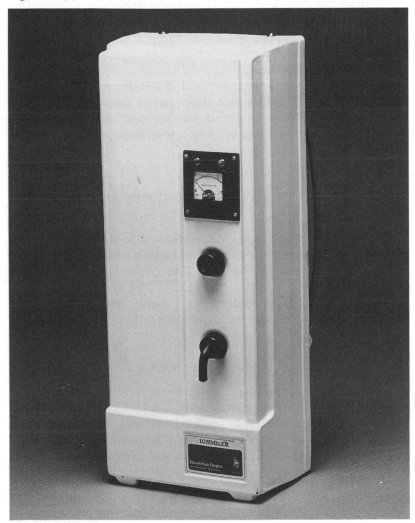

Fig. 12.10(b)   Portable de-ionizer

SELF TESTING

1. What is the purpose of shampooing?
2. Name a solvent used in wig cleaning.
3. What are the ingredients of a dry powder shampoo? Suggest reasons why this type of shampoo might be used.
4. Why is it important to know the position of stop taps in a salon water supply?
5. In what ways may water be heated for salon use?
6. Why do water pipes sometimes burst if the water in them freezes?
7. Why should a chipped shampoo basin be replaced?
8. What is the purpose of the trap under a shampoo basin?
9. What is meant by hard water?
10. Name the chemical substances which cause (a) temporary hardness (b) permanent hardness.
11. Why should purified water be used in a steamer?
12. Name two methods by which water can be purified.
13. What is the difference between purified water and soft water?
14. What is the effect on hair of using a soap shampoo if the water is hard?

TYPES OF DETERGENTS

The power of the detergent to clean surfaces depends on the presence of a **hydrophilic** (water-loving) **head** and a long **hydrophobic** (water-hating) **tail** in the detergent molecule. The hydrophilic head may have an electrical charge.

There are several types of detergents: anionic detergents, cationic detergents, ampholytes, and non-ionic detergents.

Anionic detergents

In soap and most of the soapless detergents used as shampoos, the hydrophilic head has a negative charge. These detergents are called anionic detergents. For example, sodium lauryl sulphate is the chemical name of one detergent sometimes used in shampoos. When it dissolves in water, some detergent molecules split into two parts called **ions**.

Sodium lauryl sulphate $\rightarrow$ sodium ion$^+$ + lauryl sulphate ion$^-$
(positively   (negatively
charged cation)   charged anion)

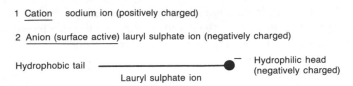

Fig. 12.11   Anionic detergent molecule

One part, the sodium ion, is small, has a positive electrical charge and is called the cation. The other part, the lauryl sulphate ion called the anion, is much larger and consists of a negatively charged head with a long tail (see Fig. 12.11). It is this part, the anion, which makes sodium lauryl sulphate a good detergent (an anionic detergent).

The structure of the anions enables the detergent to lower the surface tension of water and to form stable emulsions between water and grease when cleaning the hair during shampooing. This detergent action will be discussed later in this chapter.

Cationic detergents

Substances in this group of detergents have a positive electrical charge on the hydrophilic head of the cation (see Fig. 12.12). They include an important group of substances called quaternary ammonium compounds or quats. The one most commonly used in hairdressing is cetrimide (cetyl trimethyl ammonium bromide).

Cetrimide

Cetrimide does not give a good lather so is not used in regular shampoos but, as it is a good antiseptic as well as a detergent, it is suitable for occasional use as a medicated shampoo. Cetrimide is damaging to the eyes so a back-wash basin is required when shampooing. It may also be used in a bowl on dressing tables for disinfection of tools, and as a conditioner in products such as cream rinses, perm lotions and

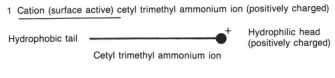

Fig. 12.12   Cationic detergent molecule

neutralizers. Anionic shampoo must be rinsed out of the hair before applying a cetrimide rinse as the negative charge on the shampoo destroys the effectiveness of the positively charged conditioner.

Ampholytes

These detergents are anionic in alkaline solutions and cationic in acidic solutions. They do not foam well so are not used alone as shampoos, but are sometimes added to shampoos as auxillary detergents to stabilize the foam and make shampoo less irritant to the eyes. **Lauryl betaine** is an ampholyte used in some shampoos as a foam booster. **Coconut imidazoline** is added to shampoos in quantities up to 20 per cent to produce very mild shampoo with low eye irritancy. **Hydroxymethyl imidazoline** in acid solution (therefore cationic and substantive to hair) is used as a restructurant in the treatment of split ends.

Non-ionic detergents

Non-ionic detergents do not ionize and the head of the molecule is neither negatively nor positively charged but still has the detergent structure of a hydrophilic head and a long hydrophobic tail. Non-ionics can be mixed with either anionic or cationic detergents. They do not give a good lather so are not used by themselves as shampoos but are added to anionic shampoos as auxillary detergents to act as foam stabilizers and conditioners. **Lauryl diethanolamide** is a non-ionic detergent often used for this purpose.

DETERGENT ACTION

Shampoos do not dissolve grease. They work by reducing the **surface tension** of water, **emulsifying** grease and keeping the grease **suspended** in water until it is rinsed away.

What is surface tension?

There are strong forces of attraction between the molecules in water. The forces at the centre of the liquid act in all directions (see Fig. 12.13) and balance each other. At the surface, however, the forces pulling the molecules inwards have practically no balancing forces acting outwards into the air. Thus the surface has an inward pull which creates surface

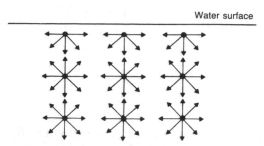

The arrows show forces of attraction
between water molecules

Fig. 12.13 Surface tension

tension, and this makes water act as though its surface has a 'skin'. The surface tension 'skin' may be demonstrated by completely filling a straight-sided vessel to the rim with water and then carefully slipping small coins down the side of the vessel into the water. The 'skin' holds the water as it rises above the surface of the vessel.

Surface tension also causes the contraction of the surface of water so that water has a tendency to form droplets and does not spread easily over surfaces.

When water is placed on a fabric it tends to remain in droplets and does not wet the fabric. For this reason water, by itself, is not a good cleansing agent. If detergent is added to a drop of water on a fabric, the water-loving heads push in between the water molecules at the surface of the drop and the water-hating tails are forced out into the air. The detergent thus expands the surface, causing the droplets to collapse, spread and wet the fabric (see Fig. 12.14). The detergent is called a **wetting agent** or surface active agent (**surfactant**).

The use of a detergent as a wetting agent can be shown by placing a few drops of water on a piece of woollen material using a dropping pipette. The water will form droplets on the surface and will not soak into the fabric. If this is repeated using water containing a little shampoo, the detergent solution will be seen to wet the fabric (see Fig. 12.15).

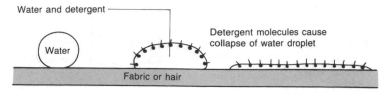

Water and detergent

Water

Detergent molecules cause
collapse of water droplet

Fabric or hair

Fig. 12.14 Lowering surface tension

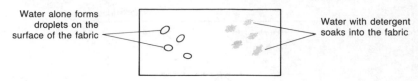

Fig. 12.15 Wetting agents

The wetting power of detergents can be compared by floating separate squares of woollen material (about 2 cm × 2 cm) on the surface of the following liquids:

- tap water
- 0.3 per cent soap solution
- 0.3 per cent sodium lauryl sulphate solution

Note in each case the time taken for the material to become wet and sink, so showing the best wetting agent. Different shampoos can also be tested in this way.

What is an emulsion?

An emulsion consists of minute droplets of one liquid suspended in another liquid. The two liquids must be insoluble in each other. All emulsions consist of two phases, the droplets forming the **disperse phase**, and the liquid in which they are suspended, the **continuous phase**. Most common emulsions consist of mixtures of oil and water. Droplets of oil suspended in water form an **oil-in-water** (O/W) emulsion, and droplets of water suspended in oil form a **water-in-oil** (W/O) emulsion. The droplets in an emulsion are large enough to be seen through a microscope (see Fig. 12.16).

The emulsion formed by shaking a few drops of oil with water soon separates into two layers. To prevent this a third substance, an **emulsifying agent** or **emulsifier** must be added so making the emulsion

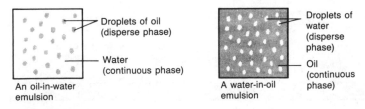

Fig. 12.16 Emulsions

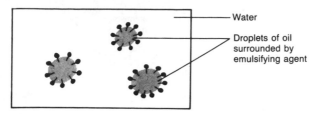

Fig. 12.17   Emulsion showing position of emulsifying agent

permanent. Detergents, lanolin, cetrimide (a cationic detergent) and synthetic emulsifying waxes such as Lanette wax (a mixture of cetyl and stearyl alcohols) act as emulsifying agents. The molecules of the emulsifying agent lower the surface tension and form a bridge between the two liquids by surrounding the droplets of the disperse phase (see Fig. 12.17).

Many cosmetic creams and lotions, such as conditioning creams and barrier cream, are emulsions. Detergent acts as the emulsifying agent for the emulsion of water and grease formed during shampooing.

HOW SHAMPOOS WORK

Detergent shampoos work in three main ways.

By acting as wetting agents

The detergent lowers the surface tension of the water so spreading the water over the surface of the hair and bringing it into closer contact with the hair.

By acting as an emulsifying agent

The anions of the shampoo molecules have negatively charged water-loving heads, and long tails which are attracted to grease. During shampooing, the tails of the anions enter the grease while the heads stay in the surrounding water (see Fig. 12.18a). The negative charges on the heads of the ions repel each other, causing the grease to roll up (see Fig. 12.18b), become dislodged from the hair and form an oil-in-water emulsion (see Fig. 12.18c). Hot water and rubbing also help to dislodge the grease from the hair. Solid particles of dirt (particulate dirt) are removed along with the grease.

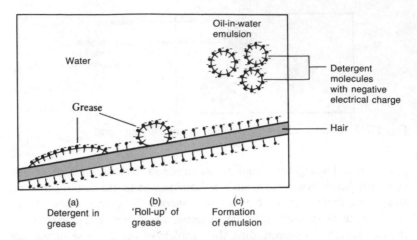

Fig. 12.18   Detergent action

By acting as suspending agents for the grease

The droplets of grease in the emulsion repel each other due to the negative charge on the detergent ions which surround the grease. Thus the droplets are prevented from joining together to form larger globules which could be redeposited on the hair. The grease remains suspended in the water until it is rinsed away.

QUALITIES OF A GOOD SHAMPOO

A good surfactant shampoo should have the following qualities:

- It should spread easily over the surface of the hair.
- A rich creamy lather should be produced. Although some detergents will clean efficiently without one, a lather is important in washing hair and skin, as it provides a concentrated solution of detergent which is easily moved over the surface of the skin or scalp. A lather also acts as a visible guide to the amount of detergent required.
- It must be a good wetting agent, yet must not make the hair so wet that it is difficult to dry out. During shampooing, hair may soak up to 30 per cent of its own weight in water. Drying must reduce that amount to the normal 10 per cent of moisture in hair.
- While being a good emulsifying agent, it should not degrease the hair and scalp excessively as this may lead to dermatitis and dry unmanageable hair.
- The shampoo should be a good suspending agent so that grease is not redeposited on the hair shafts.

Table 12.1 Comparison of the properties of soap and soapless shampoos

Soap shampoo	Soapless shampoo
Alkaline so roughens the cuticle; pH = 8–9	Neutral so leaves the hair smoother than soap shampoos; pH = 7
Forms a scum with hard water	No scum with hard water
Decomposed by acids	Unaffected by acids, so used in acid shampoos
Insoluble in salt solution	Salt is used to thicken these shampoos
May become rancid	Unlikely to become rancid
Rarely causes dermatitis	Often causes dermatitis
Better suspending power	Better wetting agents. Better removal of grease. May degrease the hair too much

- It should be easily rinsed out of the hair.
- The hair should be left manageable and lustrous when dry.
- The shampoo should not irritate the eyes or skin by being either too acid or too alkaline.

SOAP SHAMPOOS

Soap for shampoos is made by boiling vegetable oils with alkalis such as potassium hydroxide in a process called **saponification** producing soft soaps such as potassium oleate. Soap shampoos are rarely used in salons as they have many disadvantages when compared with soapless shampoos (see Table 12.1).

MANUFACTURE OF SOAPLESS SHAMPOOS

Most soapless detergents used as shampoos are based on vegetable oils such as coconut oil which is treated with sulphuric acid. There are three main types: Sulphonated oils, sulphated lauryl alcohols, and sodium lauryl ethersulphate.

Sulphonated oils

These oils, such as sulphonated castor oil, are used in conditioning shampoos. They act as an oil and a detergent at the same time and are

Table 12.2 Preparation of shampoos

	Alkali		Surfactant	Properties of surfactant
Lauryl hydrogen sulphate	+ sodium hydroxide	→	sodium lauryl sulphate	A white paste used in cream shampoos; not suitable for clear shampoos as it is not very soluble in cold water
Lauryl hydrogen sulphate	+ ammonium hydroxide	→	ammonium lauryl sulphate	A thick amber liquid
Lauryl hydrogen sulphate	+ triethanolamine	→	triethanol amine lauryl sulphate (TLS)	A thin colourless liquid; very mild Used in clear liquid shampoos
Lauryl hydrogen sulphate	+ monoethanol amine	→	monoethanol amine lauryl sulphate	Thicker than TLS, so easier to apply; mild

easily rinsed off the hair. Their manufacture is represented by the following equation

Castor oil + sulphuric acid → sulphonated castor oil
(also called Turkey Red oil)

A typical oil shampoo contains

Sulphonated castor oil 15 per cent
Sulphonated olive oil 15 per cent
Water 70 per cent.

Sulphated lauryl alcohols

These form the largest group of shampoos. Lauryl alcohol is obtained from coconut oil, and is then treated with sulphuric acid to form lauryl hydrogen sulphate. Neutralization by various alkalis gives a range of neutral surfactants used as shampoos.

Lauryl alcohol + sulphuric acid = lauryl hydrogen sulphate

The preparation and properties of various surfactants made from lauryl hydrogen sulphate is shown in Table 12.2.

Sodium lauryl ethersulphate

Some shampoos are based on sodium lauryl ethersulphate, which is milder than sodium lauryl sulphate and, being more soluble in cold water, is suitable for clear shampoos as well as cream shampoos.

FORMULATION OF SOAPLESS SHAMPOOS

Soapless shampoos are available in several forms. Some actually contain small quantities of added soap, not to increase the amount of detergent but only to thicken the shampoo.

Clear liquid shampoos

These may contain triethanolamine lauryl sulphate, ammonium lauryl sulphate, or sodium lauryl ether sulphate. An example is

Triethanolamine lauryl sulphate 20 per cent
Coconut monoethanolamide 2 per cent (improves lather)
Water 78 per cent
Perfume and colour traces.

Liquid cream shampoos

These are similar to clear liquid shampoos but are thickened by the addition of soap, which makes the shampoo opaque.

Solid cream shampoos

These contain

Sodium lauryl sulphate   25 per cent
Soap   5 per cent
Water   70 per cent.

Gel shampoos

These contain 20–25 per cent of triethanolamine lauryl sulphate thickened with methyl cellulose to a semi-solid, jelly-like consistency.

Aerosol shampoos

Sodium lauryl sulphate and triethanolamine lauryl sulphate may be dispensed as an aerosol foam. These detergents, however, are corrosive to metals so the aerosol container is often made of glass with a plastic outer cover. Sodium lauryl sarcosinate is less corrosive and is therefore more frequently used. The shampoo foams as it leaves the container due to the propellent gas passing through the detergent solution.

Additives

Additives to soapless shampoos include the following:

- **Perfumes** to give the shampoo a pleasant smell. Most perfumes are made synthetically but some are obtained from plant oils known as essential oils.
- **Colour** to increase the visual appeal of the product.
- **Thickeners** such as sodium alginate, soap, or common salt. Note that a shampoo which is thick is not necessarily concentrated.
- **Preservatives**, e.g. formaldehyde or Nipagin, to prevent bacterial growth in shampoo.
- **Foam stabilizers** such as lauryl diethanolamide (a non-ionic detergent).

MODIFICATION FOR SPECIAL PURPOSES

Hairdressers are increasingly using general purpose shampoos for all types of hair and dealing with particular problems afterwards by use of conditioning creams, lotions and other products. However, many shampoos are designed for special pupuses or to treat particular conditions. Although the full range of shampoos may not be used in the salon, some may be available for sale to clients, and hairdressers should be able to offer advice regarding the home use of all kinds of shampoo. The type and amount of shampoo base (the detergent which forms the bulk of the shampoo) may be varied or additions may be made to the shampoo base. The most common shampoo bases are triethanolamine lauryl sulphate and ammonium lauryl sulphate as these work well in acid-based shampoos. Most modern shampoos are made slightly acid by the addition of citric acid or lactic acid.

Greasy hair

For greasy hair the percentage of soapless detergent in the shampoo is increased from the 15−20 per cent used in shampoos for normal hair to as much as 50 per cent. Lemon and lime shampoos are often associated with greasy hair but there is no scientific advantage in such shampoos.

Dry hair

There are several alternatives for dry hair:

- The percentage of soapless detergent in the shampoo may be as low as 10 per cent to make the shampoo less degreasing.
- Oils such as olive oil, coconut oil and almond oil may have been added to the shampoo base to increase the amount of oil on the hair.
- A sulphonated oil shampoo which acts as an oil and detergent at the same time is useful on dry hair.
- Lanolin (wool fat similar to sebum) may be added to the shampoo base, though some people are allergic to it. Jojoba, a liquid wax from the seeds of a shrub grown mostly in Mexico, is also similar to sebum and may be added instead of lanolin.
- Other conditioners, including beer, egg and various herbs, may be added to shampoos but often in such small quantities as to have little effect. Beer is best used as a final rinse when it stiffens the hair slightly.

Frequent use

Frequent use shampoos are intended for those who prefer to shampoo every day or alternate days. To avoid dryness of the hair these shampoos must not be too de-greasing and so have a low detergent content of only about 10 per cent.

Extra mild

Extra mild shampoos with a very low eye irritancy and containing up to 20 per cent of coconut imidazoline are used as baby shampoos or for very delicate or damaged hair. Because sebum is not produced until a child is about 4 years old, these shampoos contain a very low percentage of the shampoo base.

Medicated

Medicated shampoos contain antiseptics to reduce the number of micro-organisms on the scalp and are useful in cases where scalp irritation (or an itchy scalp) leads to scratching, possibly to be followed by infection. These shampoos are not intended as anti-dandruff shampoos as they do not reduce scaling. The shampoo may be cationic (a cetrimide shampoo), or anionic with an added antiseptic.

Cationic

Cationic detergent shampoos (cetrimide shampoos) are useful because cetrimide is an antiseptic as well as a detergent and is substantive to hair. The antiseptic film remains on the hair even after rinsing. This type of shampoo does not give a good lather but is useful as an occasional treatment shampoo. A back-wash basin is recommended when using a cetrimide shampoo because cetrimide is damaging to the eyes.

Anionic with antiseptics

Most medicated shampoos have an anionic shampoo base (usually a lauryl sulphate) to which antiseptics such as hexachlorophane or trichloro-carbanilide are added. The addition of coal tar to the shampoo base is useful for the treatment of psoriasis.

Anti-dandruff

Anti-dandruff shampoos are designed to reduce the scaling which causes dandruff; they contain about 2−3 per cent of zinc pyrithione (zinc omadine) usually in a lauryl ether sulphate base. Selenium sulphide (2−5 per cent) may be used but sometimes gives rise to dermatitis.

Brightening

Brightening shampoos are used to give highlights to brown hair or to revive blonde hair which has darkened with age. The most effective contain 3 per cent of hydrogen peroxide added to a soapless shampoo base. Camomile, a vegetable dye obtained by infusion of dried camomile flowers, is sometimes added to a shampoo base as a brightener and gives slight yellow tones to blonde hair.

Colour

Colour shampoos may be formulated by the addition of temporary dyes (azo dyes), semi-permanent dyes or vegetable dyes to a soapless shampoo base. The use of vegetable dyes has increased recently: both henna, used to give red colour to black hair, and walnut, used to revive the colour of dark brown hair, are available.

Protein

Protein shampoos do not contain protein itself but protein hydrolysates, including individual amino acid molecules, dipeptides (two amino acids chemically combined) or short chains of amino acids in a shampoo base. They are used on damaged hair particularly after perming, bleaching or tinting. The protein hydrolysates are substantive to hair so have a conditioning effect, making the hair smoother and adding lustre. Many of the amino acids will cling to the outside of the hair shaft but on damaged hair which is more porous, some will enter the cortex and build up new but weak linkages. Split ends may be made to cling together but there is no permanent repair.

Conditioning

Conditioning shampoos designed to be used as a shampoo and conditioner in one, and avoid the necessity to use a cream rinse after shampooing, contain silicone oils (dimethicone) which coat the hair with a fine, soft, protective film.

Acid balanced

Acid balanced shampoos are designed to keep the hair in its natural acid state, or to return hair to that state after alkaline treatments such as perming, bleaching and tinting. The swelling of the hair shaft caused by alkalis is reduced, the cuticle is left well aligned and its surface smooth. Acid balanced shampoos also help to stop loss of colour from tinted hair by keeping the cuticle scales flat during shampooing. The shampoo base is usually ammonium lauryl sulphate. The pH of the shampoo is usually adjusted to 4.5–5.5 by the addition of citric acid but this makes the shampoo more irritant to the eyes.

Lacquer removing

Lacquer-removing shampoos containing spirit (alcohol) are used to dissolve shellac-based lacquers on the hair. More modern lacquers contain plastic resins which are soluble in water and will wash out with a normal shampoo. The lacquer-removing shampoo should be applied before wetting the hair so that the lacquer is dissolved first.

Safety notes

- Wipe up any spilled shampoo immediately: it can be very slippery.
- Take care not to let shampoo enter the client's eyes. If necessary, wash shampoo from the eyes with plenty of tepid water.
- Avoid shampoo dermatitis by removing rings before shampooing, rinsing and drying the hands well afterwards, and using hand creams at night.

pH VALUES

The pH values of shampoos are shown in Fig. 12.19.

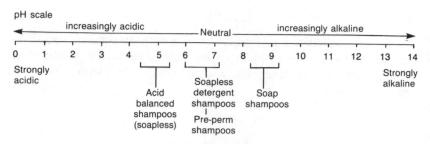

Fig. 12.19 pH values of shampoos

SELF TESTING

1. Describe the structure of a detergent molecule.
2. What is meant by an anionic detergent?
3. Name one cationic detergent and describe its uses.
4. What is meant by an auxillary detergent? What are the uses of such detergents?
5. What is meant by surface tension?
6. Why is a detergent called a wetting agent?
7. What is meant by an oil-in-water emulsion?
8. How does a detergent clean hair?
9. What are the qualities of a good shampoo?
10. What are the disadvantages of soaps used as shampoos?
11. Name two substances often used as soapless shampoo bases.

12. What are the ingredients of (a) brightening shampoos (b) colour shampoos?
13. What is meant by (a) an acid balanced shampoo (b) a protein shampoo? For what purposes would they be used?
14. For what type of lacquer is a lacquer-removing shampoo required? What is the active ingredient of a lacquer-removing shampoo?

13

SETTING AND DRYING

The changes involved in curling or waving straight hair, or straightening curly or wavy hair, can be brought about in two ways:

- **physical changes** involving the mechanical shaping of the hair, producing a temporary set
- **chemical changes** to the structure of keratin producing a permanent set (see Chapter 14).

TEMPORARY SETTING

Temporary setting can be carried out as a **cohesive set** on wet hair as in roller setting and in blow waving using a hand dryer, or as a **temporary heat set** on dry hair using heated curling tongs or crimping irons. In both cases the process is a physical change involving only a change in the shape of the keratin molecules. No chemical change takes place, no new substances are formed, and the change is easily reversed. This can be contrasted with permanent waving, which gives a permanent set requiring chemical changes to the structure of keratin. It is, however, the chemical structure of keratin and the elasticity of the hair which enables temporary setting to take place.

ELASTICITY OF HAIR

Hair is elastic due to the coiled spring structure of the keratin in the cortex of the hair (see Fig. 13.1), which allows the hair to stretch and to spring back to its original length when released. The scales of the cuticle slide over each other to allow the hair to stretch. The amount

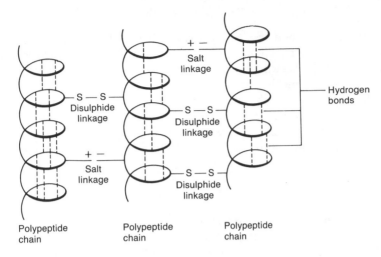

Fig. 13.1 Keratin showing numerous hydrogen bonds

of stretching is limited by the hydrogen bonds which hold the coils of the spring together, for although they are weak they are very numerous.

Keratin

Keratin in unstretched hair is known as **α-keratin** (alpha-keratin). If the hair is stretched, some of the hydrogen bonds are broken and the spiral structure straightens out to form **β-keratin** (beta-keratin). When the stretching force is removed α-keratin is re-formed. The change on stretching is called the α–β transformation of keratin and is reversible. (Alpha is the first letter of the Greek alphabet and beta the second.)

$$\begin{array}{c} \text{extended} \\ \alpha\text{-keratin} \xrightarrow{\hspace{4cm}} \beta\text{-keratin} \\ \text{(unstretched hair)} \xleftarrow{\hspace{4cm}} \text{(stretched hair)} \\ \text{released} \end{array}$$

If hair is stretched with sufficient force, a point is reached when the hair will no longer return to its original length when the force is removed. The hair has then reached its **elastic limit**. When stretched beyond this limit a sudden extension of the hair may take place due to the breaking of a large number of hydrogen bonds. If the stretching force is again increased the hair eventually breaks, due to the breaking of the polypeptide chains.

Tensile strength

The force or tension needed to break a hair is known as its tensile strength. Dry hair stretches by a third to a half of its original length before breaking. Wetting hair increases its elasticity as water enters the hydrogen bonds, enabling them to extend further, but the tensile strength is reduced so that it breaks more easily. The water in the hydrogen bonds is known as **bound water**. The amount of bound water is greater if hair is steamed and the hair may then be stretched by as much as twice its original length and will still spring back if the stretching force is removed.

Demonstrating tensile strength

The stretching power of a hair and the breaking point can be shown using the apparatus shown in Fig. 13.2.

Use as long a hair as possible and gradually increase the number of small weights (5 or 10 grams at a time) on the hair, supporting the weight in the hand at each addition to prevent a sudden increase in tension. Note the length of the hair after each addition, allowing the hair to stretch for several minutes between additions. Note the number of grams required to break the hair. This is a measure of its tensile strength. Repeat the process several times using different hairs to obtain an average. Try also both wet and dry hairs. Typical results are shown in Table 13.1.

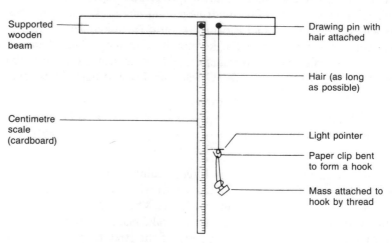

Fig. 13.2 Elasticity of hair

Table 13.1 Typical results for dry hair

Original length (cm)	Length on breaking (cm)	Amount of stretch (cm)	$\dfrac{\text{Stretch}}{\text{Original length}}$	Weight causing causing breakage (grams)
18	24	6	$\frac{6}{18} = \frac{1}{3}$	90
20	26	6	$\frac{6}{20} = \frac{1}{3}$ approx.	80
27	40	13	$\frac{13}{27} = \frac{1}{2}$ approx.	100

COHESIVE SET

This type of set is carried out on wet hair by roller setting, blow waving, finger waving and during pin curling.

A good long-lasting cohesive set may be achieved if:

- The hair is in good condition and so is sufficiently elastic.
- Tension is applied to the wet hair to stretch it into the desired shape, e.g. by winding tightly round rollers or by use of a brush in blow waving or by a comb in finger waving.
- The hair is thoroughly dried while still being stretched under tension. If rollers are removed before the hair is properly dry there will be some loss of set. On completion of drying the hair will remain set in its new position even when the stretching force is removed.
- Setting and dressing aids are used to help to control the entry of moisture into the set hair.

What happens during setting

The setting of hair depends on its ability to stretch, so that hair which is over-processed or very dry does not take a good set due to lack of elasticity. The stretching of dry hair is limited by the hydrogen bonds, and to obtain a greater extension setting is carried out on wet hair. Water molecules enter the hydrogen bonds between the coils so allowing the hair to stretch further. Stretching is achieved by winding the hair tightly on rollers, or by the movement of the brush in blow drying.

The hair is dried in this stretched state and the water held in the hydrogen bonds is evaporated off. Because the hair is still under tension, the hydrogen and oxygen atoms of the original hydrogen bonds may be

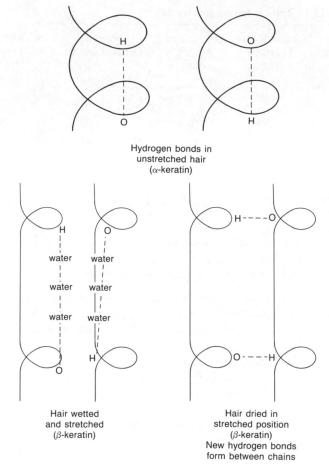

Fig. 13.3   Cohesive set

too far apart to rejoin. New hydrogen bonds will form in a different position along the chain or between two adjacent polypeptide chains (see Fig. 13.3). The hair is thus set in the β-keratin position and does not spring back to its original position when the rollers are removed. The α-keratin or unstretched state returns whenever the hair becomes wet again, and the set is thus lost.

Demonstrating a cohesive set

Make a bundle of about 12 hairs of equal length (the longer the better, but not less than 20 cm) and knot them together at each end. Suspend

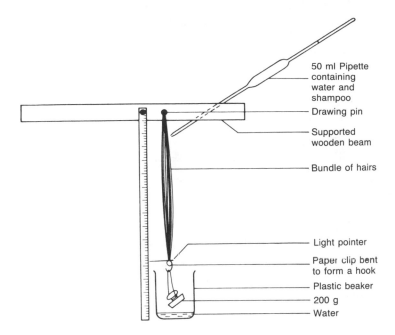

50 ml Pipette containing water and shampoo

Drawing pin

Supported wooden beam

Bundle of hairs

Light pointer

Paper clip bent to form a hook

Plastic beaker

200 g

Water

Fig. 13.4 Demonstration of cohesive set

the hair as shown in Fig. 13.4 and measure the length between the knots. Stretch the hairs by adding a mass of 200 g. With a 50 ml pipette, run hot water containing a little shampoo down the hairs until they are thoroughly wet. Allow time for the hairs to stretch and then note the new length. Remove the stretching force and dry the hair with a hand dryer. Note that the hair returns to its original length. Stretch the hair again, wetting it as before. Now dry the hair with the 200 g still in position, removing it only when the hair is perfectly dry. Note that the hair now remains at its stretched length. The hair as been set. Wet it with cold water and the hair will return to its original length.

Preserving the set

A cohesive set is easily destroyed if the hair becomes damp. Hair itself is hygroscopic, and the moisture absorbed from a damp atmosphere is sufficient to convert β-keratin back to α-keratin. Thus in Britain the normal humidity of the air gradually destroys the set, though in very dry areas of the world a cohesive set will last for long periods. The absorption of moisture is reduced by the natural surface coating of sebum and by applying conditioning creams, setting lotions and hair spray.

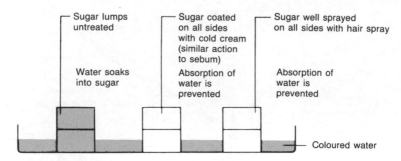

Fig. 13.5   Action of sebum and hair spray

It is important that the air in the salon itself should not be excessively humid, or the set may be destroyed before the client leaves the salon! A wall hygrometer should be used to indicate the level of humidity in a salon (see Chapter 2) and humidity should be controlled by good ventilation.

Demonstrating the action of sebum and hair spray

Obtain six cubes of sugar. Cover two cubes on all sides with cold cream to produce a similar effect to sebum. Cover two more with a coating of hair spray. Leave the remaining two cubes untreated. Place the cubes in a shallow layer of coloured water as shown in Fig. 13.5. Note that the water rises in the untreated cubes, but is prevented from rising by the cold cream and hair spray.

HAIR DAMAGE DURING COHESIVE SETTING

- Use of spiked rollers for setting may cause splitting of the hair shafts.
- Frequent use of brush rollers or very tight rollers may cause traction alopecia (hair loss by pulling) especially at the front margin.
- Careless use of a blow dryer may cause scalp burns and cicatrical alopecia.
- The hair cuticle may be damaged if the hot nozzle of a blow dryer is allowed to touch the hair. The dryer should be kept moving to avoid overheating any area.
- Frequent brushing of wet hair as in blow drying may damage the cuticile by abrasion, and is more damaging than dry brushing. Silicone setting lotions help to prevent this. The air flow from the dryer should also be from roots to points of hair to keep the cuticle as flat as possible.

TEMPORARY HEAT SET

Setting of dry hair by electrically heated tongs, crimping irons, hot brushes, marcel waving irons or heated rollers is best carried out soon after the hair has been shampooed and dried, because the amount of internal moisture in the hair is then greater. Heat setting reduces the moisture content of the hair, and if frequently repeated may lead to loss of condition and dry, brittle hair.

The hair is both heated and stretched at the same time. The higher the temperature, the more water is removed from the hair and the greater the number of hydrogen bonds broken. New hydrogen bonds are formed in a different position on the polypeptide chain to set the hair in the desired position. The new bonds are completely destroyed by hot water but only slightly by cold. Hot water is therefore required to break the set.

HAIR DAMAGE DURING HEAT SETTING

- Repeated heating may raise or break the scales of the cuticle, making the hair rough and therefore lacking in lustre. The hair may dry out leading to static electricity on brushing and combing.
- Burns to the scalp or damage to the hair cuticle can result if tongs, etc., are too hot. A comb placed between the tongs and the scalp helps to prevent burns.

SETTING AIDS

These include setting lotions, mousses, and gels.

Setting lotions

Setting lotions are used by sprinkling the lotion evenly over the towel dried hair immediately before roller setting. They prevent the hair from drying out too quickly during the setting process and, after the hair is dried, they form a clear flexible film around the hairs. This film helps to preserve the life of the set by preventing atmospheric moisture from entering the hair shafts.

Gum setting lotions

Older types of setting lotions contained natural gums which, when added to a mixture of alcohol and water, formed a thick sticky solution or mucilage. The gums were obtained by damaging the bark of certain trees, enabling the gum to ooze out and be picked off by hand. The most common were **gum tragacanth** from Turkey and **gum karaya** from India. On the hair, the gum left a brittle film which tended to flake off easily.

Plastic setting lotions

Modern setting lotions contain 1–2 per cent of plastic resins dissolved in a mixture of alcohol and water. A thin flexible film of plastic resin is left on the hair after evaporation of the alcohol and water during drying.
  There are two main resins used:

- **Dimethyl-hydantoin formaldehyde (DMHF):** this is soluble in water and in alcohol and is easily washed from the hair. The film is glossy but brittle and plasticizers such as glycerol or dimethyl phthalate are added to soften the film.
- **Polyvinyl pyrrolidone (PVP):** this is substantive to hair, is antistatic, and gives the hair a soft feel by being a humectant so attracting moisture to the hair. This hygroscopic quality has the disadvantage that the film becomes soft and sticky. To overcome this difficulty polyvinyl acetate (PVA) is usually added to PVP (in the proportion of 40 parts PVA to 60 parts PVP). This gives a firmer hold and is more resistant to humidity.

Coloured setting lotions

These are a popular form of temporary colour which washes out at the first shampoo. Acid dyes (azo dyes) are joined chemically to PVP/VA resins which are dissolved in water and alcohol.

Heat-styling setting lotions

Lotions designed for use during blow drying often contain protein hydrolysates and silicone oils as conditioners, in addition to plastic resins. Silicone oils give the hair a smoother surface and so lessen friction between the hair and the brush. They also produce a heat resistant film which helps to prevent hair damage by the hot blow dryer nozzle. It is important to use lotions specially designed for blow drying as setting lotions intended for roller setting make the hair too sticky to work with during blow drying.

Mousses

These contain plastic resins and silicone oils in a detergent solution of water and alcohol which produces a foam of very small bubbles when released from a pressurized aerosol container. An auxillary detergent such as methyl thiazolinone (an ampholyte) is used to give a foam which soon breaks down on the hair and leaves a coating of silicone and plastic resin. Mousses of different strengths are available according to the hold required. The addition of silicones, which are resistant to heat, make mousses suitable for use during blow drying and with heated styling appliances. Mousses can also be formulated with azo dyes to give a temporary colour.

Gels

Gels are greaseless products containing plastic resins with a plasticizer in the gel base. They are thixotropic, that is they are thick as they leave the tube or other container but become liquid when rubbed into the hair. Gels have a strong moulding power and some can be used to make the hair stiff as in punk styles.

Self Testing

 1. Name two types of temporary sets.
 2. What is meant by (a) elasticity (b) tensile strength?
 3. Describe the bond structure of hair keratin.
 4. Why is hair elastic?
 5. Is hair stronger when wet or when dry?
 6. Which bonds limit the stretching of hair?
 7. What is meant by (a) α-keratin (b) β-keratin?
 8. What is 'bound' water and what effect does it have on hair?
 9. How can a long-lasting cohesive set be obtained?
10. Why can a good set never be obtained on dry over-processed hair?
11. What is meant by temporary heat setting and what type of appliances may be used to produce this type of set?
12. What damage to hair can be caused by (a) incorrect blow drying (b) temporary heat setting?
13. Name three types of setting aids.
14. What is the purpose of using a setting lotion?
15. What are the main ingredients of (a) gum setting lotions (b) plastic setting lotions (c) heat-styling setting lotions?

Hair Drying

The final drying of hair may be carried out using a salon hood dryer, a hand blow dryer or an infra-red dryer, the water being removed by evaporation in each case. A hood-type dryer is used after roller setting and the dried hair is then dressed out into the desired style. Blow drying involves first blotting the hair with a towel to absorb sufficient water to prevent dripping, then simultaneously setting and drying the hair to its completed style, using a brush and blow dryer. Infra-red dryers are useful in cases where movement of the hair during drying is undesirable.

Towel drying

Towel drying is usually carried out immediately after shampooing to absorb surplus water, but still leaving the hair sufficiently wet to allow the hair to stretch easily during setting. A towel consists of loosely woven cotton threads between which are narrow air spaces. Water is drawn up into these air spaces by a surface tension effect known as **capillary rise**. Water is also absorbed into the fibres of the towel itself.

During towel drying, the hair should be blotted rather than rubbed so avoiding physical damage to the cuticle by friction.

Drying by evaporation

During evaporation water changes from a liquid into water vapour. Hair dryers are designed to provide conditions for the rapid evaporation of moisture from the hair. Evaporation depends on the following conditions: temperature, humidity and surface area.

Temperature

Evaporation can take place at any temperature but occurs more rapidly as the temperature rises. Heat energy from the hair dryer is absorbed by the molecules of water making them move faster and enabling them to escape into the air more quickly from the surface of liquid water. The greater the heat, the faster the molecules move and the greater the evaporation.

Humidity

If the air surrounding a wet head is saturated with moisture the air can hold no more, and no evaporation takes place. The hair dryer fan normally removes moist air from around the wet head allowing evaporation to take place quickly. If the cooler air entering the dryer from the salon is humid the drying process will be slower. The effect may be avoided by good salon ventilation.

Surface area

Evaporation takes place faster when a large area of hair is exposed to the air. Thus hair dries more quckly by blow drying when the hair is constantly being spread out by the brush, than if it is wound on rollers and dried under a hood dryer.

Hood dryers

These are used to dry hair after roller setting. They may be wall mounted, arranged in banks as seating units, or be single pedestal dryers which can be moved into position as desired. They consist basically of an electric motor which turns a fan, so blowing cold air over an electrically heated element. The power of hood dryers varies from 500 to 2000 watts. In some hood dryers the electric motor and heating element are enclosed in the hood itself. In seating units a more powerful heater and motor are placed behind the seating arrangement, the hot air being ducted to the hood (see Fig. 13.6).

Temperature control

The working temperature of the dryer is now usually controlled by a variable resistance switch (see Fig. 13.7). (Resistance is a measure of

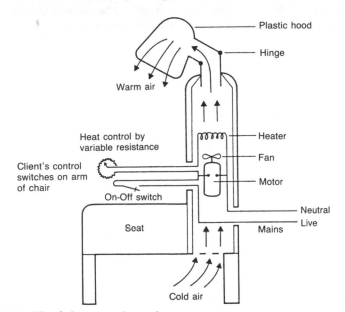

Fig. 13.6 Hood dryer: seating unit

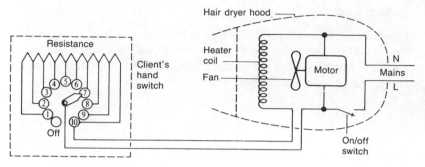

Fig. 13.7 Variable resistance switch

the ease or difficulty with which an electric current flows through a wire.) The switch may be on the arm of the seating arrangement and controlled by the client, or on the dryer hood and controlled by the hairdresser. When in position 1 the electricity goes through a long length of wire (offering a high resistance) which cuts down the current in the heating element, so the working temperature is low. If the pointer is at 10 the length of resistance wire is short and the current is greater so making the dryer hotter. Some dryers also have an adjustable automatic timer switch which switches off the current after a set time. The time of drying depends on the amount of the hair. Fine hair should be dried at a lower temperature than coarse hair. The hair should be allowed to cool before removing rollers, clips or pins or the set will drop slightly.

Safety notes

- Never operate switches with wet hands.
- To avoid overheating the dryer, never cover any air vents while the dryer is in use.
- Never place metal clips or pins close to the client's scalp as they become hot under the dryer and may cause burns.

Blow dryers

These depend on air being blown over a heated electrical element by a fan in the same way as in hood dryers. The power is usually between 500 and 1200 watts. The air flow speed and the working temperature can be controlled by switches on the dryer handle. The air flow can also be adjusted by use of a nozzle or by a diffuser (see Fig. 13.8). Nozzles are used to concentrate the flow of air when drying small sections of hair.

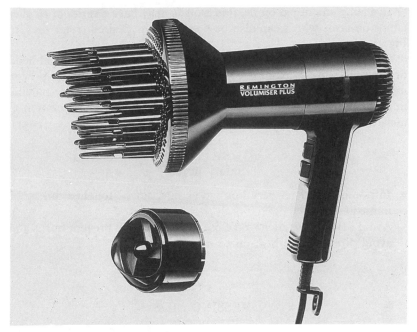

Fig. 13.8 Blow dryer and attachments

Diffusers have the opposite effect to a nozzle and slow down the flow, dispersing the air over a wider area with less disturbance of the style. Diffusers are often used for drying permed hair into scrunch styles. A filter is fitted over the air intake at the back of the dryer to prevent dust from collecting in the motor. This filter must be regularly cleaned or the air intake would be reduced and cause overheating of the dryer element.

Safety notes

- Never use a hand-held dryer near a water supply or with wet hands.
- Always make sure the filter is clean.
- Always keep the dryer moving so as not to burn the hair or scalp.

Infra-red dryers

Infra-red dryers, sometimes called **accelerators**, were introduced for drying precision-cut hair to avoid disturbing the style. Hand models are available containing a 275 watt infra-red lamp. Stand models have three or five lamps mounted on flexible arms or may have a series of smaller lamps on arms which can also be positioned as desired (refer back to Fig. 11.3).

The lamps are more comfortable for the client than traditional hood dryers and noise is eliminated. More recently **rollerballs** have been introduced in which the source of infra-red heat is constantly moving to avoid 'hot spots'. In all cases drying takes place by evaporation of moisture.

Safety notes

- Infra-red lamps get very hot and should not be touched during or immediately after use.
- Avoid placing the client too close to the lamps to prevent burns and avoid directing the heat on to the client's eyes.

DRESSING AIDS

These include control creams or dressing creams, mousses, gels, brilliantines and hair sprays, all of which are used on dry hair.

Control creams

Control creams (dressing creams) are used in very small quantities on dried hair but before dressing out, to replace sebum removed by shampooing. They reduce static electricity on dry hair, keep the hair in place, and as oil increases the reflection of light, control creams add lustre to the hair. They help to preserve the set by preventing the entry of moisture into the hair shafts. The creams are water-in-oil emulsions containing a very small proportion of water as they are used on dry hair and must not spoil the set. The oil may be vegetable oil such as castor oil or almond oil, but is more usually a mineral oil (a light paraffin oil).

Mousses

Mousses similar to those used on wet hair as setting aids may be used on dry hair to promote curl for scrunch styles.

Gels

Gels may be greaseless products containing plastic resins with a plasticizer, or contain a fixative such as propylene glycol in alcohol and water thickened with methyl cellulose, to give a gel consistency. Clear micro-gel preparations are oil-in-water emulsions in which the oil is dispersed as sub-microscopic particles giving a less greasy feel than ordinary oil-in-water control creams.

Brilliantines

Brilliantines may be in liquid or solid form used after setting and drying, or in spray form used after dressing is complete. They impart gloss and help to preserve the set. Liquid brilliantines consist of mixtures of light mineral oil (liquid paraffin oil) and castor oil or almond oil with added perfume. Solid brilliantines contain mixtures of paraffin oils and soft paraffin thickened by paraffin wax or carnuba wax (obtained from the surface of palm leaves). For spraying from an aerosol can, they contain castor oil dissolved in methylated spirit. A fine oily film is left on the hair when the spirit evaporates. The sprays are sometimes known as **hair gloss** or shine, and should be applied sparingly.

Hair spray

Hair sprays, or lacquers as they were previously known, are applied to the hair from aerosol containers after dressing is complete. They keep the hair in position and help to preserve the set by preventing absorption of moisture from the air.

A good hair spray should

- dry quickly leaving a tough, clear, flexible film
- be neither tacky in a humid atmosphere nor flake off in a dry atmosphere
- be easily washed from the hair
- be non-irritant to the skin.

Shellac-based lacquer

True lacquers contained shellac, a natural resin produced by the female lac insect of India or Malaysia, which was dissolved in alcohol. This is now rarely used as it leaves a stiff film on the hair. It is also insoluble in water so needs a lacquer-removing shampoo containing borax or alcohol to dissolve the film from the hair.

Plastic resin hair spray

Modern hair sprays contain 4–6 per cent of plastic resins dissolved in alcohol. PVP/PVA or DMHF resins like those in setting lotions, or acrylic resins may be used. Silicone oils are added to give a good spread over the hair and to add sheen. Cetrimide or lanolin may be added as conditioners, and isopropyl myristate as a plasticizer to soften the film. Hair spray aerosols should be held about 20 cm (8 inches) from the head while spraying.

Firmness of hold

The firmness of the hold of a hair spray depends on:

- the type of resin
- the concentration of the resin
- the degree of plasticizing.

Sunscreen spray

Sunscreen sprays contain para-aminobenzoic acid as an additive to prevent sun damage and bleaching of hair by ultra-violet rays (see the section on Weathering in Chapter 9).

Safety notes

- Use a shield to protect the client's eyes and contact lenses if worn.
- Avoid inhaling hair spray fumes and use in a well-ventilated area.
- Keep hair spray off the skin as some (e.g. those containing lanolin) can cause dermatitis.
- The solvents in hair sprays are flammable, so do not spray near naked flames or hot electrical appliances.

AEROSOLS

A wide variety of hairdressing preparations including shampoos, setting mousses and hair sprays are produced as aerosols. In addition to the main ingredients of the product, the aerosol also contains a **propellant** which

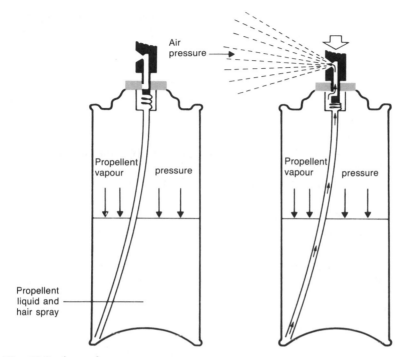

Fig. 13.9 Aerosol can

forces the product out of the can when the nozzle is pressed (see Fig. 13.9). The propellant is as highly volatile liquid (often propane or butane) so easily turns to a vapour at room temperature. The vapour always fills the space above the product in the can and creates a pressure on the surface of the liquid. When the can is opened to the atmosphere by pressing the nozzle, the pressure of the vapour inside the can pushes the liquid contents of the can out because its pressure is much greater than that of the outside air. The vapour pressure inside the can remains the same whether the can is full or nearly empty, so that the spray comes out of the can at the same pressure throughout the life of the aerosol.

Type of spray

The fineness and type of spray is determined by the size and shape of the opening in the nozzle. In the case of shampoos and mousses which contain detergents, the product foams as it leaves the can. Some of the liquid propellant also leaves the can, vaporizes and expands, so bubbling through the detergent solution creating a foam as it passes out into the air. In mousses the foam is designed to break down quickly on the hair.

Safety notes

- Propane and butane propellants are highly flammable and care must be taken not to spray near a naked flame or any hot surface.
- Store aerosols in a cool place: heat increases the pressure in the can by making more liquid turn to vapour, so that the can may explode if overheated.
- Never place empty cans on a fire. They will still contain vapour and may explode.
- Do not puncture a can even if you think it is empty. It may still contain vapour and liquid which would spray out with considerable force.
- If the nozzle becomes blocked, try holding it under running hot water for a few seconds. Never try to pierce the nozzle.
- Read the manufacturer's instructions before use and always follow them.

MIRRORS

Hairdressers use the dressing-table mirror in front of the client when cutting, setting, blow drying and dressing the hair, and a hand mirror to show the client the back of the head.

Mirrors are made of sheets of glass coated on one side with silver. The use of mirrors depends on the properties of light. We can see an object only if light travels from that object to our eyes. The light takes the shortest path, that is, it travels in a straight line between the object and the eye. The law—light travels in straight lines—is the basis of the use of mirrors and of the diagrams drawn to indicate the pathway of rays or beams of light. When a beam of light strikes a mirror surface, the light is reflected regularly so that the light comes away from the surface at the same angle as that at which it strikes the mirror (see Fig. 13.10).

The path of the reflected light when using a back mirror is shown in Fig. 13.11. The hairdresser adjusts the hand mirror by experience to obtain the correct angles of reflection. It should be moved first to one side then the other across the back of the head so that the client can see the whole of the back. If the hair is very long the client may not be able to see the full length in the small hand mirror so must turn her back towards the dressing-table mirror and adjust the hand mirror at an angle to see the style in the larger mirror.

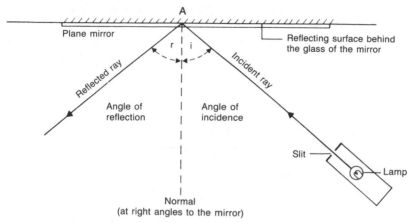

Fig. 13.10 Reflection of light

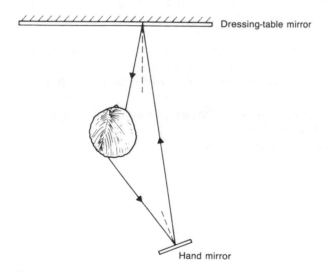

Fig. 13.11 Use of a back mirror

Lateral inversion

Your client may startle you by saying 'Oh, are you left-handed?' when you are busy cutting with scissors in your right hand. Or if you have a new ring on your right hand she may ask 'Have you become engaged?' She does this when looking through the mirror on the dressing table in front of her. A mirror appears to turn an object round so that the right side of the object appears as the left side of the image. This is known as lateral inversion.

The effect of lateral inversion can easily be shown if you stand in front of a mirror and hold your left ear with your left hand. In the mirror your image or reflection will appear to be holding the right ear with the right hand.

SELF TESTING

1. What is meant by (a) capillary rise (b) humidity?
2. What is evaporation and what conditions affect the speed at which it takes place?
3. Describe the working of a hand dryer. What is the purpose of using (a) a nozzle (b) a diffuser?
4. What safety precautions should be taken in using (a) a hood dryer (b) a hand dryer (c) an infra-red dryer?
5. What are the advantages of using an infra-red dryer?
6. What is the purpose of using (a) dressing creams (b) hair spray?
7. What are the ingredients of modern hair spray?
8. What safety precautions should be taken in the use and disposal of aerosol containers?
9. How, using mirrors, would you ensure that clients with long hair could see the back of their hair?
10. What is meant by lateral inversion?

14

PERMANENT WAVING

The reasons for natural curliness or straightness of hair are not fully understood. It was at one time thought that wavy hair had an oval cross-section, straight hair a round cross-section, and very tight curly hair a kidney-shaped cross-section but this has been discounted. Another theory is that straight hair grows from a straight follicle and a curly hair grows from a curved or spiral follicle (see Fig. 14.1).

It is more probable that curl is caused by a difference in structure between one side of the cortex of a hair compared with the other, giving rise to a **'para' cortex** and an **'ortho' cortex** (see Fig. 14.2).

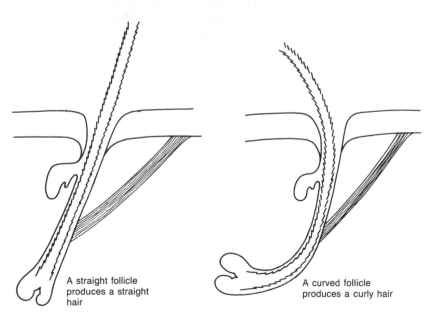

A straight follicle produces a straight hair

A curved follicle produces a curly hair

Fig. 14.1 Effect of follicle shape

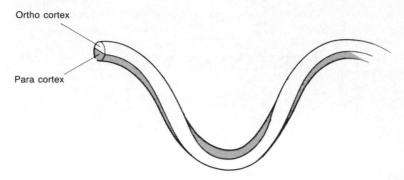

Fig. 14.2 Ortho cortex and para cortex

The ortho cortex has a less dense structure and is always on the outside of the wave. The structure may be compared to the wave of permed hair in which the outer curve is stretched (therefore less dense) and the inner surface of the wave compressed (this will be shown in Fig. 14.5).

PERMANENT SETTING

During permanent waving the amount of curl in the hair is altered chemically by changing the internal structure of the hair shaft. The hair is given a permanent set which cannot be removed by wetting with either hot or cold water.

PROCEDURE BEFORE PERMING

Examine hair and scalp

Examine the hair and the skin of the scalp. No perm should be given if there are signs of infection or if cuts, abrasions or inflammation of the skin are present. Very slight skin defects may be covered with vaseline or collodion.

Consult client

Consult the client about the type of perm required and about previous salon and home treatments. Refer to the client's record card if available.

Check condition

Make sure that the hair is in good enough condition for satisfactory perming and that there are no incompatible chemicals already present on the hair. Tests for elasticity, porosity and incompatibility are described in Chapter 10.

Shampoo hair

Shampoo the hair using a clear soapless shampoo with a pH of 7 and without additives such as lanolin which may affect penetration of the perm lotion. Shampooing removes sebum, lacquer and other hairdressing products which may create a barrier to the entry of perm lotion into the cortex.

Towel dry hair

Towel dry the hair. If the hair is too wet the perm lotion will be diluted, and if too dry the perm lotion may be too strong for the hair.

Do a pre-perm test

Note the amount of any previous perm left in the hair. Shampooing will make this obvious as any straightening effect of setting or blow drying will be removed. Perming for a second time over already permed hair is inadvisable and could lead to serious chemical damage. Cutting may be necessary to remove a small amount of previous curl remaining near the points of the hair.

Read instructions

Read the manufacturer's instructions for use of both the perm lotion and neutralizer. These instructions should always be followed.

Apply pre-perm filler

If the porosity varies along the hair shaft, a pre-perm filler may be beneficial. The filler contains protein hydrolysates which cling electrostatically to amino acid groups both on the cuticle and in the cortex of the hair and will even out porosity. The filler is applied to the towel

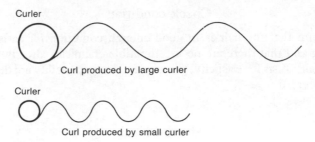

Fig. 14.3 Size of curl

dried hair after shampooing and left on the hair during perming. Again read the instructions, as protein hydrolysates are added to some perm lotions by manufacturers and the pre-perm lotion is then unnecessary.

Choose lotion

Decide on the type and strength of lotion required according to hair condition, previous treatment, and intended hair style.

Choose curlers

Decide on the size of curler to be used. The diameter of the curler determines the final curl size. Larger curlers produce larger curls or waves; smaller curlers make smaller waves (see Fig. 14.3).

Make test curls

As a precautionary measure, a series of test curls can be made if there is uncertainty about hair condition and the possible success of the perm, or if there is doubt about the strength of lotion or size of curlers required. Using several small sections near the crown, wind and process each section as in normal perming using different sized curlers or different strengths of lotion, then neutralize and rinse. Examine and assess the result. Test curls are essential before attempting to perm bleached hair.

STAGES IN PERMANENT WAVING

Permanent waving takes place in two distinct stages: application of perm lotion and application of neutralizer.

Application of perm lotion

The perm lotion is applied to hair which has been wound on to curlers or rods. A reducing agent (a substance which gives hydrogen to another substance during a chemical reaction) in the lotion breaks some of the cystine linkages in keratin. This softens the hair and enables it to take the shape of the curler.

Application of neutralizer

On the application of the neutralizer (sometimes called the normalizer or the oxidizer), an oxidizing agent (a substance which gives oxygen or takes hydrogen away during a chemical reaction) in the neutralizer enables the cystine linkages to be rebuilt in new positions along the polypeptide chains, thus holding the hair in the desired curly or waved shape.

The chemical reactions involved in perming are explained in detail later in this chapter.

TYPES OF PERM LOTIONS

There are two main types of perm lotions: alkaline and acid.

Alkaline perm lotions

Alkaline perm lotions with a pH of 9.5 are available in different strengths for use on different types of hair, but are particularly suitable for hair which is in good condition or coarse hair which is hard to perm.

Acid perm lotions

Acid perm lotions with a pH of 6−7 are gentler than alkaline perms, and are often preferred for use on fine hair which is easy to process or hair which has been previously permanently coloured or bleached.

INGREDIENTS OF PERM LOTIONS

Reducing agent

A reducing agent is the main ingredient of perm lotions. Its purpose is to break down some of the cystine linkages of the hair.

In alkaline lotions the reducing agent ammonium thioglycollate is most commonly used, as follows:

- a 10 per cent solution for non-porous or resistant hair
- an 8 per cent for normal hair in good condition
- a 5−6 per cent solution for fine hair, bleached or tinted hair.

Monoethanolamine thioglycollate is an alternative reducing agent used mainly because it has a less objectionable smell.

In acid lotions the reducing agent is often glyceryl monothioglycollate. A 15 per cent solution of ammonium thioglycollate (stronger than in alkaline lotions) is sometimes used but at a lower pH than in alkaline lotions.

Swelling agent

A swelling agent in the lotion raises the cuticle scales and allows easy penetration of the lotion into the hair.

In alkaline lotions ammonium hydroxide is the swelling agent giving the lotion a pH of 9.5.

In some acid lotions with a pH of 6 the swelling agent is omitted and heat is applied during processing by use of a hair dryer or infra-red heater. The heat raises the cuticle scales. In other acid lotions, urea and urease are added to the reducing agent immediately before application to the hair. A controlled amount of ammonium hydroxide is produced from the urea to make the hair swell and aid penetration of the lotion but the pH remains low (7 or less).

Wetting agents

Wetting agents, e.g. alkanolamides (non-ionic detergents), are included in perm lotions to lower the surface tension and bring the lotion into closer contact with the hair.

Conditioners

Conditioners include protein hydrolysates, particularly if the lotion is intended for use on bleached or tinted hair. This avoids the need for a pre-perm filler. In '**moisturizing**' perms for dry hair, humectants such as glycerol or polyvinyl pyrrolidone are added to attract moisture to the hair.

Thickeners

Thickeners are used to produce a cream which keeps in position on the hair better than a watery lotion. Mineral oils with cetyl alcohol as an emulsifying agent form a stable emulsion which does not break down easily on the hair. The oil remains in the emulsion and is not deposited on the hair shaft where it would delay penetration of the reducing agent.

Perfume

Perfume is included to improve the smell of the lotion. Masking the smell of ammonium thioglycollate is difficult as the reducing agent tends to break down the perfume.

INGREDIENTS OF NEUTRALIZERS

The neutralizer may be a cream or liquid type. The main ingredient is always an oxidizing agent such as hydrogen peroxide or sodium bromate.

Cream neutralizers

Cream neutralizers consist of an oil-in-water emulsion which is mixed with 20 volume (6 per cent) hydrogen peroxide immediately before use.

Liquid neutralizers

Liquid neutralizers contain a 5 per cent solution of sodium bromate with 1 per cent of soapless detergent to produce a foam which holds the neutralizer in place on the hair. Unlike hydrogen peroxide, sodium bromate is effective in acid solutions. For use after alkaline perm lotions, citric acid or acetic acid may be added to sodium bromate neutralizers to give a pH of 4. This neutralizes any alkali left in the hair and leaves the cuticle smoother.

SELF TESTING

1. What are the reasons for curliness in hair?
2. What is meant by a permanent set?

3. State the pH value of (a) alkaline perm lotion (b) acid perm lotion.
4. For what types of hair are acid perms particularly suited?
5. What are the ingredients of an alkaline perm lotion? State the use of each ingredient.
6. What are the ingredients of (a) cream neutralizer (b) liquid neutralizer? What is the purpose of a neutralizer?
7. How and why would you carry out (a) a test for porosity (b) an elasticity test (c) an incompatibility test?
8. What type of shampoo should be used before perming?
9. Why should hair be towel dried before perming?
10. What does a pre-perm lotion contain? Why would a pre-perm lotion be used?
11. What effect has rod diameter on the finished curl?
12. Why should test curls be made before perming? How are these carried out?

CHEMICAL ACTION DURING PERMING

Action of perm lotion

The hair is treated with perm lotion either before or after winding small sections of hair on to rods or curlers. Winding should be without tension because the hair is in a delicate state during perming and is easily broken. The perm lotion contains a **reducing agent**, that is a chemical which gives hydrogen to another substance during a chemical reaction. During perming the hydrogen atoms from the reducing agent break some of the disulphide bonds in the cystine linkages of keratin by adding themselves to the sulphur atoms. This splits the cystine molecules and each forms two cysteine amino-acid molecules (see Fig. 14.4). This chemical reaction involving the addition of hydrogen is called reduction. About 20 per cent of the cystine linkages in hair are broken in alkaline perms but only about 10 per cent in acid perms, making acid perms more suitable for use on damaged hair or hair that is easy to process.

Heat may be required to assist the penetration of the lotion and to speed the chemical reaction. In alkaline perms, the added ammonium hydroxide aids penetration, and sufficient heat for satisfactory processing is produced if the hair is enclosed in an insulating plastic perm cap to retain the heat of the scalp. In acid perms, urea is sometimes added to aid penetration but often mild heat is required either from a hair dryer or infra-red heater, both to aid penetration and to speed processing.

The breaking of the cystine linkages enables the hair to take the shape of the rods by movement of the polypeptide chains in relation to each

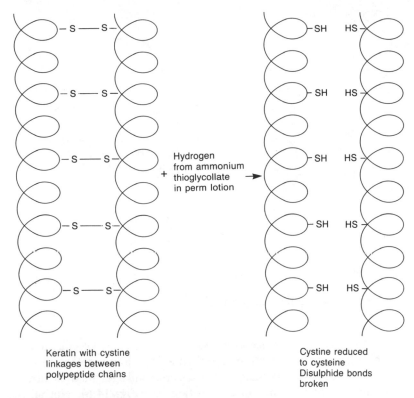

Keratin with cystine
linkages between
polypeptide chains

+ Hydrogen
from ammonium
thioglycollate
in perm lotion →

Cystine reduced
to cysteine
Disulphide bonds
broken

Fig. 14.4 Process of reduction during perming

other (see Fig. 14.5). The firmness of the curl depends on the strength
of the lotion and the processing time. When a satisfactory curl has been
achieved (carry out curl tests until the S-shape of the curl has the same
diameter as the curler), the lotion must be rinsed from the hair to stop
further reduction, but the curlers must be kept in position until the
completion of the oxidation process which follows. The hair is blotted
dry with a towel to remove excess water before neutralizing.

Action of neutralizer

Neutralizing is carried out to make the newly curled shape permanent,
by rebuilding the disulphide bonds in a new position on the polypeptide
chains. This is a process of oxidation, that is a chemical reaction in which
oxygen is added to a substance. The neutralizer contains an oxidizing
agent usually either hydrogen peroxide or sodium bromate. Oxygen from

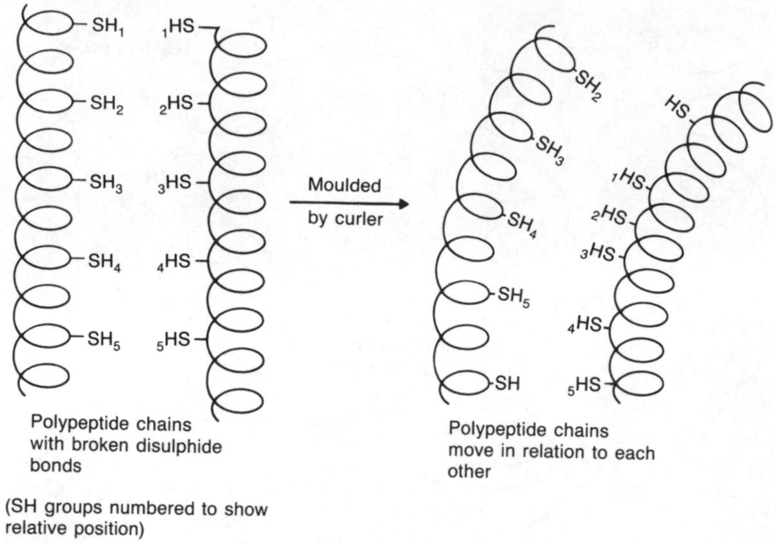

Fig. 14.5 Moulding the hair to the shape of the curler

the oxidizing agent combines with hydrogen in cysteine molecules to form water. Adjacent sulphur atoms are then able to join together to make new disulphide bonds. Permanent cystine cross linkages are thus formed, so setting the hair in the curled position (see Fig. 14.6). Not all the sulphur atoms are suitably placed to link with a second sulphur atom, so fewer cross linkages are re-formed than were originally present. Perming therefore always results in some weakening of the hair.

Note

Neutralizing a perm is an oxidation process and not true chemical neutralization, which is the reaction between an acid and an alkali to form a salt.

Length of processing time

Processing time for perm lotion

The length of processing time for the perm lotion has to be judged by the hairdresser with the help of **curl tests** (see Chapter 10). Processing time depends on:

- The **porosity** of the hair: the more porous the hair the quicker the reaction.

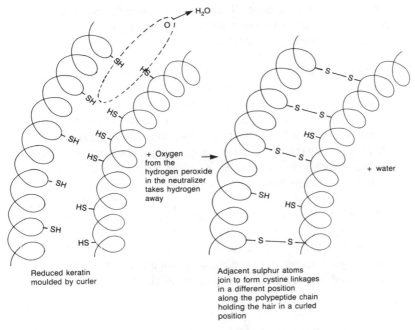

Fig. 14.6 Oxidation to rebuild disulphide bonds

- The **strength** of the perm lotion: the stronger the lotion the faster it will act.
- The **pH** of the lotion: the higher the pH, the quicker the reaction.
- **Temperature:** heat speeds chemical reactions. Processing will be faster if the salon temperature is high, or if a hair dryer or an infra-red heater is used. The client's body heat can increase the speed of processing if the head is covered with an insulating perm cap.

Processing time for neutralizer

The length of processing time for the neutralizer depends entirely on the manufacturer's instructions. Two-thirds of the neutralizer is usually added before the rods are removed and this is left for about 5 minutes (according to instructions). After the rods are removed the remaining one-third is applied, and left for several minutes before rinsing the neutralizer from the hair.

Safety notes

- To avoid dermatitis, protective gloves should always be worn when applying perm lotion.

- The lotion should be kept off the client's skin as far as possible during perming. Barrier cream or vaseline may be applied around the ears and hair line before perming, but care must be taken to prevent contact of the cream with the hair itself.
- Remember that hair, skin and nails are all keratin: perm lotion softens hair and so it will also affect skin and nails.
- The hair should not be pulled or wound too tightly as perm lotion weakens hair and breakages may occur. Avoid twisted rubbers on perm curlers which may cut into hair and cause breakage.
- Pull burns may result if tension on the hair allows perm lotion to enter the hair follicles. Scratching this irritation may lead to infection known as folliculitis. Breakage of the hair inside the follicle may occur.
- Avoid allowing perm lotion to enter the client's eyes. If this happens rinse immediately with plenty of tepid water. Use a back-wash basin if possible when rinsing perm lotion from the hair.
- Ammonium thioglycollate reacts with iron to form a purple coloured compound. Contact between perm lotion and any iron object should be avoided to prevent discolouration of the hair.

TREATMENTS AFTER PERMING

Acid rinses

After alkaline perming, acid rinses (pH restorers) with a pH of about 4 may be useful to neutralize alkali left in the hair and reduce any roughening of the cuticle. Ascorbic acid is often used as it is a reducing agent (or anti-oxidant) as well as an acid and is effective in stopping further oxidation. Acids also help to stop the loss of soluble oxidation products formed from hair protein during perming.

Substantive conditioners

Substantive conditioners of the cetrimide type are useful after perming, as they are taken up to a greater extent if the hair is damaged and remain effective even after rinsing.

Colour

Perming hair which has been previously permanently coloured leads to some loss of colour, because permed hair is more porous and some colour may wash out. Natural colour may also be lightened by oxidation during neutralizing. This slight loss can be overcome by use of a matching temporary or semi-permanent colour after perming.

EFFECTS OF UNDER-PROCESSING OR OVER-PROCESSING

Perming is a balance between the number of disulphide bonds broken by reduction and the number reformed by oxidation during neutralizing.

Under-processing

Under-processing during reduction means that too few bonds are broken and a new wave shape cannot be achieved.

This may be due to:

- lack of penetration of the perm lotion due to grease or other substance on the cuticle
- use of an incorrect lotion (too weak) for the type of hair
- insufficient processing time
- coldness of the surroundings.

Over-processing

Over-processing during reduction means that too many bonds are broken for neutralizing to be completely effective. The hair would be weakened and would not hold its shape.

This may be due to:

- use of a strong perm lotion on porous hair
- over-long processing time
- excessive temperature.

Under-neutralizing

Under-neutralizing means that insufficient disulphide bonds would be rebuilt in the correct positions and the intended curl would be lost.

This may be due to:

- omitting the neutralizing process
- not leaving the neutralizer on the hair long enough
- removing the curlers before neutralizing was complete.

Over-neutralizing

Over-neutralizing results in loss of cross linkages. Excessive oxidation changes the amino acid cystine into cysteic acid which will not form cross linkages. The number of disulphide bonds may thus be considerably reduced resulting in lack of curl and weakening of the hair.

This may be due to:

- leaving the neutralizer on too long
- using too strong an oxidizing solution.

HAIR DAMAGE DURING PERMING

Loss of cystine linkages

Loss of cystine linkages always takes place during perming but the effect is increased by incorrect processing. Loss of linkages results in a reduction of elasticity and tensile strength.

This may be caused by:

- over-processing (reduction) during perming if more bonds are broken than can be repaired by neutralizing
- over-neutralizing, because excessive oxidation may change cystine to cysteic acid which does not form linkages.

Loss of soluble protein material

Loss of soluble protein material from the hair results in the weakening of the internal hair structure. This may be caused by over-oxidation and lack of suitable conditioning after processing.

Cuticle damage

Damage to the cuticle may result from fragments of cuticle scales breaking off due to the swelling of the hair during perming.

Hair breakage

Hair breakage may be caused by

- tension applied to the hair during perming through winding the hair too tightly on the curlers, the curler elastic pressing on the hair or the elastic being twisted over the curl

- lotion entering hair follicles through tension on the hair: inside the follicle the hair is in a soft state and the extra warmth of the follicle may be sufficient to increase the speed of reaction and break the hair
- perming hair previously weakened by bleaching.

pH VALUES

The pH values of products used in perming are shown in Fig. 14.7.

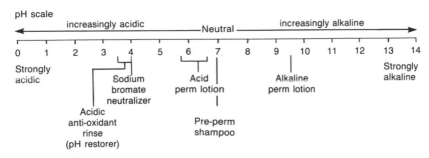

Fig. 14.7 pH values of products used in perming

SELF TESTING

1. Describe the chemical reaction that takes place when perm lotion is applied to hair.
2. What is the name of the amino acid formed when the disulphide bonds are broken by chemical reduction?
3. What percentage of disulphide bonds are broken by (a) alkaline perms (b) acid perms?
4. What is the purpose of a perm cap?
5. Describe the chemical process which takes place during neutralizing.
6. How does neutralizing in perming differ from chemical neutralization?
7. Why does perming always weaken hair?
8. What factors affect the speed of processing?
9. Why should perms always be wound without tension?
10. What is meant by a pull burn? What effect may a pull burn have on the hair and skin?
11. What precautions should be taken to protect the skin of both the client and hairdresser during perming?

12. Why does tinted hair sometimes lose colour during perming? What can be done to compensate for this loss?
13. What is the cause and effect of (a) under-processing a perm (b) under-neutralizing?
14. Describe the possible causes of hair damage in permed hair?

15

COLOURING HAIR

Natural hair colour depends on the type and amount of pigment contained in the cortex of the hair. This pigment is introduced into the growing hairs by colour-producing cells called **melanocytes** at the base of the hair follicles.

The pigments in hair are

- black and brown pigments or **melanin**
- red and yellow pigments or **pheomelanin**.

Mixtures of these pigments are responsible for all hair colours from blonde (mostly red and yellow pigment) through red, light and dark brown to black. Failure of melanocytes to produce pigment results in white hair. Grey hair is considered to be a mixture of white and coloured hairs rather than as a hair colour itself.

Albinism is due to a rare defect in which melanocytes in all parts of the body fail to produce pigment. This results in white skin, white hair and lack of colour in the iris of the eyes. A person suffering from this defect is known as an **albino**.

WHAT IS COLOUR?

When we talk about the colour of an object we normally mean its colour as seen in daylight, that is in light from the sun. Natural daylight is referred to as '**white light**', but in fact it can be split into a band of seven colours as shown in the **spectrum** (see Fig. 15.1) or as seen in a rainbow. For practical purposes indigo is now often omitted as it is hard to distinguish from violet.

The molecules of a pigment or dye in an object absorb certain colours of light and reflect others. The colours which are reflected to our eyes determine the colour we 'see'.

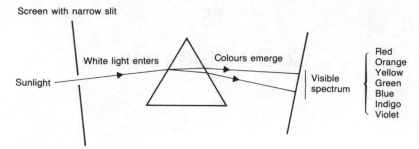

Fig. 15.1 The spectrum

- A red object reflects red light to our eyes and absorbs the other colours.
- A blue object reflects blue light and absorbs the other colours.
- A white object reflects all the colours of the spectrum and absorbs none.
- A black object absorbs all the colours and reflects none.

EFFECT OF ARTIFICIAL LIGHTING

Colour may appear to change if an object is viewed under different colours of light. Thus the colour of hair and clothing as seen under yellow 'sodium' street lighting may look quite different from their colour in daylight. As the spotlights at a disco change colour, so does the apparent colour of the clothes and hair of the dancers.

Choosing salon lighting

The appearance of hair may thus be affected by the colour of the light produced by salon lighting. The effect of predominantly red and blue lights on various heads of hair is shown in Fig. 15.2. It is important in a salon to have artificial lighting with a colour mix as near as possible to that of daylight. Tungsten filament lamps (ordinary electric light bulbs) give a light with more red and less blue than daylight. This makes blue pigments darker (blacker) and red colours deeper (redder). White fluorescent lighting has less red and more blue than daylight, and makes blue pigments appear deeper and red pigments darker. **'Warm white' fluorescent tubes** give the nearest match to daylight and are to be preferred for salon use in areas used for hair colouring. (See also the section on salon lighting in Chapter 2.)

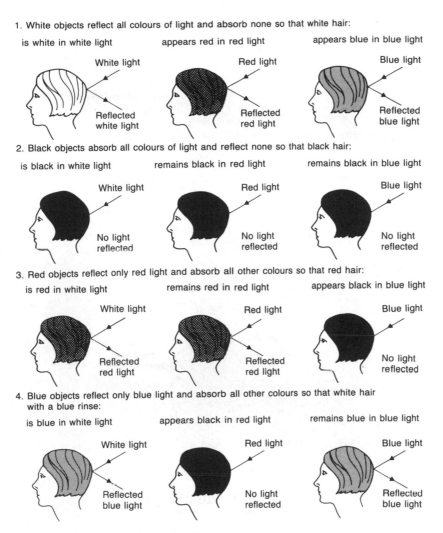

1. White objects reflect all colours of light and absorb none so that white hair:

   is white in white light   appears red in red light   appears blue in blue light

2. Black objects absorb all colours of light and reflect none so that black hair:

   is black in white light   remains black in red light   remains black in blue light

3. Red objects reflect only red light and absorb all other colours so that red hair:

   is red in white light   remains red in red light   appears black in blue light

4. Blue objects reflect only blue light and absorb all other colours so that white hair with a blue rinse:

   is blue in white light   appears black in red light   remains blue in blue light

Fig. 15.2 Effect of red and blue light on hair colour

Effect of coloured ceiling and walls

The ceiling and walls of a salon should not be too deeply coloured as light reflected from them may affect the colour of objects in the room (see Fig. 15.3). The most suitable colour is white as there is little absorption of light, and no effect on colour.

Dark walls absorb light energy, and more light will have to be provided than if the walls have a light coloured finish with a good reflecting surface.

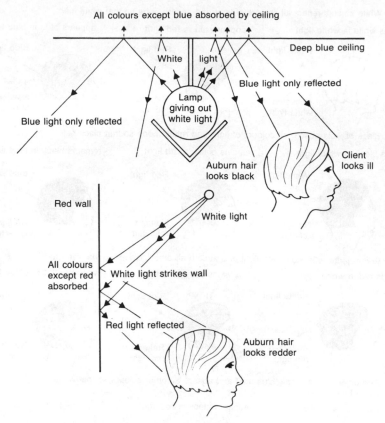

Fig. 15.3 Effect of coloured ceiling and walls

MIXING PIGMENTS

In practice, pigments rarely reflect one single spectrum colour, but reflect varying amounts of a band of adjacent spectrum colours. Omitting indigo, which is hard to distinguish from violet, the order of colours in the spectrum is red, orange, yellow, green, blue and violet. Thus a yellow pigment normally reflects orange and green in addition to yellow, while a blue pigment also reflects a little green and violet (see Fig. 15.4). If yellow and blue pigments are mixed, the only colour reflected by both is green, since the mixture strongly absorbs the other spectrum colours (see Fig. 15.5).

Adding red pigments to the mixture of yellow and blue will result in

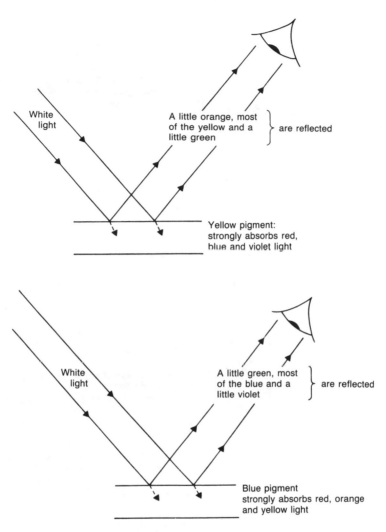

Fig. 15.4 Reflection of light by pigments

the absorption of the green (see Fig. 15.6). No colour will therefore be reflected, and so the mixture produces black. This is only true if the pigments in the mixture are present in the correct proportion. Different proportions of the three pigments may produce brown or grey. Manufacturers obtain many shades of brown in semi-permanent and temporary dyes by mixing red, blue and yellow pigments in different proportions.

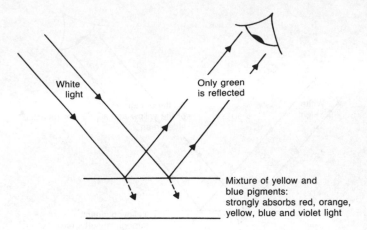

Fig. 15.5   Mixing yellow and blue pigments

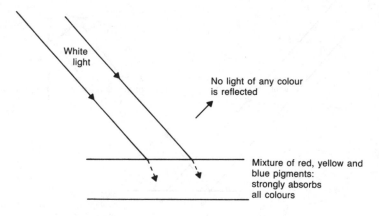

Fig. 15.6   Mixing red, yellow and blue pigments

In the mixing of pigments the colours red, yellow and blue are often called the primary colours because they cannot be made by mixing other colours. Secondary colours are made by mixing two primary colours. For example:

$$Red + yellow = orange$$
$$Red + blue = violet$$
$$Blue + yellow = green$$

SEPARATING COLOURS

The colours in some hairdressing products, for example plastic setting lotions, can be separated by use of **chromatography**.

Make up a solvent containing:

butanol	100 ml
0.880 ammonia	1 ml
water	44 ml
ethanol	20 ml

Place 50 ml of this solvent in a Shandon chromatography tank. Drop a spot of each of six different colours of setting lotions on a chromatography paper (25 cm × 25 cm) about 2 cm from the bottom of the paper as shown in Fig. 15.7. Clip the sides of the paper together to form a cylinder, and stand the paper in the solvent inside the tank, ensuring that the spots of dye are above the level of the solvent. The solvent travels up the paper by capillary rise, separating the colours in the setting lotions due to differences in their solubility. The most soluble of the mixture of dyes will travel highest up the paper. If a Shandon tank is not available, strips of chromatography paper may be suspended from a cork in a measuring cylinder or boiling tube. When separation has taken place, allow the paper to dry in a fume cupboard. Note the colours produced from each dye. Brown dyes will be found to consist of various proportions of the three pigments red, blue and yellow.

CORRECTING COLOURS

Adding colour to the hair may result in the development of unwanted colours, particularly if the hair is blonde and contains yellow pigment,

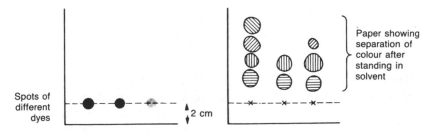

Fig. 15.7   Separation of colours by chromatography

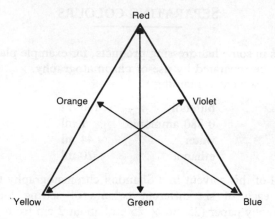

Fig. 15.8 The colour triangle

or if the hair is grey and contains a mixture of coloured and white hairs. Consider the effect of adding auburn (red) dye to various types of hair. Added to brown hair, the dye would produce an acceptable red-brown, but added to blonde (yellow) it would result in orange (yellow + red = orange). Similarly, added to grey hair (a mixture of light brown and white) the brown would become red-brown (acceptable) but white would become red (unacceptable).

Adding a blue rinse or an ash colour which may contain blue pigment to blonde (yellow) hair may give rise to an unwanted green cast (blue + yellow = green). The unwanted colour may be corrected by the addition of a small quantity of a suitable pigment which will absorb the offending colour. Thus a little red pigment will absorb green, or a green dye (some ash shades contain green pigment) will absorb red.

A colour triangle of the spectrum colours is shown in Fig. 15.8, and is useful as an aid to colour correction. The offending colour may be corrected by addition of the colour opposite to it in the colour triangle.

COLOURING AND DE-COLOURING

Hair colouring is achieved by the application of a pigment or mixture of pigments to the hair. Unless bleaching is taking place at the same time, colouring involves the addition of a dye to the natural pigment of the hair. Thus the natural colour must be taken into account before adding any colour.

Removal of the natural colour or bleaching is a chemical reaction which changes the pigments of hair into colourless compounds inside the hair shaft. The chemical reaction involves the addition of oxygen to the pigment and the process is called oxidation.

Both permanent colouring and bleaching require the use of hydrogen peroxide as an oxidizing agent.

HYDROGEN PEROXIDE

Strength of hydrogen peroxide

For salon use, hydrogen peroxide is available in various **volume strengths** from 10 volume to 100 volume. The volume strength is the number of parts of free oxygen obtainable from one part of hydrogen peroxide. Thus:

1 part of 20 volume hydrogen peroxide gives 20 parts of free oxygen

or

1 ml of 20 volume hydrogen peroxide gives 20 ml of free oxygen

or

1 ml of 100 volume hydrogen peroxide gives 100 ml of free oxygen.

The strength of hydrogen peroxide may also be expressed as the percentage of pure hydrogen peroxide in the solution. The **percentage strength** is the number of grams of hydrogen peroxide in 100 grams of solution. Thus a 30 per cent solution contains 30 g of hydrogen peroxide, and therefore 70 g of water in 100 g of solution. As 1 ml of 30 per cent solution of hydrogen peroxide gives 100 ml of free oxygen, a 30 per cent solution is equivalent to a 100 volume strength solution. The percentage strengths corresponding to other volume strengths are calculated by proportion.

$$100 \text{ volume strength} = 30 \text{ per cent solution}$$
$$10 \text{ volume strength} = 3 \text{ per cent solution}$$
$$20 \text{ volume strength} = 6 \text{ per cent solution}$$
$$30 \text{ volume strength} = 9 \text{ per cent solution}$$
$$40 \text{ volume strength} = 12 \text{ per cent solution}$$
$$60 \text{ volume strength} = 18 \text{ per cent solution}$$

The volume strength of hydrogen peroxide can be measured by a special type of hydrometer called a **peroxometer** (see Fig. 15.9). The hydrometer is floated in hydrogen peroxide and the volume strength read directly on the scale at surface level.

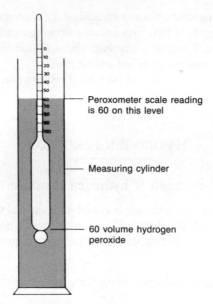

Peroxometer scale reading is 60 on this level

Measuring cylinder

60 volume hydrogen peroxide

Fig. 15.9 Use of a peroxometer

Properties of hydrogen peroxide

Colourless liquid

Hydrogen peroxide is a colourless liquid. (Cream peroxides are used by some hairdressers. These are not pure hydrogen peroxide and have added conditioners. They cannot be diluted accurately in the same way as liquid hydrogen peroxide.)

Oxidizing agent

Hydrogen peroxide is an oxidizing agent as it gives oxygen to other substances during chemical reactions. Concentrated hydrogen peroxide may break the polypeptide chains in hair keratin by oxidation so causing breakage of the hair shaft. It also causes skin burns: 40 volume hydrogen peroxide is the strongest solution which can be applied to hair without damage.

In hairdressing, hydrogen peroxide is used

- as an oxidizing bleach (20—30 volume for normal bleaching and 40 volume for bleached tips)
- for the oxidation of permanent dyes (10—30 volume)
- as an oxidizing agent in neutralizer after perming (20 volume).

Easily decomposed

Hydrogen peroxide is easily decomposed into water and oxygen by the following:

- alkalis such as ammonium hydroxide (ammonia)
- heat from the sun or radiators
- sunlight
- dust
- copper, lead or iron compounds
- organic substances such as blood.

Effect of acids

Acids (pH 3–5) prevent the release of oxygen from hydrogen peroxide and small quantities of salicylic or phosphoric acid are often added during manufacture to stabilize the peroxide and prevent premature release of oxygen during storage.

Storage of hydrogen peroxide

Hydrogen peroxide is easily split into water and oxygen and should be protected during storage from substances and conditions which lead to its decomposition.

- Storage should be in a cool dark place, in a dark brown bottle or an opaque plastic container.
- An air space should be left over the liquid to allow oxygen to accumulate without danger of bursting the container.
- Storage bottles should be smooth on the inside, as any projection forms a point at which decomposition begins.
- As with other chemicals, hydrogen peroxide once poured out should not be returned to the bottle.
- Hydrogen peroxide, though not itself flammable, assists fire by giving off oxygen when heated. Consequently it should not be stored near flammable liquids such as alcohol or hair sprays.
- Hydrogen peroxide should be stored in relatively small quantities to prevent deterioration during its shelf-life. The more concentrated the peroxide, the more liable it is to lose its strength.

Dilution of hydrogen peroxide

If the correct volume strength of hydrogen peroxide is not available it is sometimes necessary to dilute a stock solution of a higher strength to obtain the required lower strength solution. Since tap water may be slightly alkaline and would therefore decompose the hydrogen peroxide, dilution should be carried out when necessary by using deionized water. The quantity of water to be added for the dilution may be calculated as shown in the following examples.

To obtain 30 volume hydrogen peroxide from 60 volume

Because 30 volume hydrogen peroxide is $^{30}/_{60}$ or ½ as strong as 60 volume, ½ the diluted solution must be 60 volume hydrogen peroxide and the remainder (½) is water.
The 30 volume solution contains equal quantities of 60 volume hydrogen peroxide and water.

To obtain 20 volume hydrogen peroxide from 60 volume

Because 20 volume hydrogen peroxide is $^{20}/_{60}$ or ⅓ as strong as 60 volume, ⅓ of the diluted solution must be 60 volume hydrogen peroxide and the remainder (⅔) is water.
The 20 volume solution contains 1 part of 60 volume hydrogen peroxide and water.

Volume strength

Dilutions by volume strength are listed in Table 15.1.

Table 15.1 Dilution of hydrogen peroxide by volume strength

Stock solution available	Required solution	Fraction stock solution required	Fraction water required	Parts stock solution	Parts water
100 vol	60 vol	$\frac{60}{100} = \frac{3}{5}$	$\frac{2}{5}$	3	2
100 vol	40 vol	$\frac{40}{100} = \frac{2}{5}$	$\frac{3}{5}$	2	3
100 vol	30 vol	$\frac{30}{100} = \frac{3}{10}$	$\frac{7}{10}$	3	7
100 vol	20 vol	$\frac{20}{100} = \frac{2}{10} = \frac{1}{5}$	$\frac{4}{5}$	1	4
60 vol	40 vol	$\frac{40}{60} = \frac{2}{3}$	$\frac{1}{3}$	2	1
60 vol	30 vol	$\frac{30}{60} = \frac{1}{2}$	$\frac{1}{2}$	1	1
60 vol	20 vol	$\frac{20}{60} = \frac{1}{3}$	$\frac{2}{3}$	1	2
40 vol	30 vol	$\frac{30}{40} = \frac{3}{4}$	$\frac{1}{4}$	3	1
40 vol	20 vol	$\frac{20}{40} = \frac{1}{2}$	$\frac{1}{2}$	1	1
30 vol	20 vol	$\frac{20}{30} = \frac{2}{3}$	$\frac{1}{3}$	2	1

Table 15.2 Dilution of hydrogen peroxide by percentage strength

Stock solution available	Required solution	Fraction stock solution required	Fraction water required	Parts stock solution	Parts water
30%	12%	$\frac{12}{30} = \frac{2}{5}$	$\frac{3}{5}$	2	3
30%	6%	$\frac{6}{30} = \frac{1}{5}$	$\frac{4}{5}$	1	4
18%	6%	$\frac{6}{18} = \frac{1}{3}$	$\frac{2}{3}$	1	2
12%	3%	$\frac{3}{12} = \frac{1}{4}$	$\frac{3}{4}$	1	3

Percentage strength

Dilutions by percentage strength are calculated in the same way (see Table 15.2).

SELF TESTING

1. Name the natural pigments of the hair.
2. From what type of cell is pigment produced? Where are these cells situated?
3. Which layer of the hair contains most pigment?
4. What is meant by albinism?
5. What is meant by 'white light'?
6. Name the colours of the spectrum.
7. Why is the colour of artificial light important in a salon?
8. What type of artificial light is best for colour work in a salon?
9. What colour of semi-permanent dye is often made by mixing red, blue and yellow dyes?
10. What colour of dye would you use to remove a green cast from a client's hair?
11. How should hydrogen peroxide be stored?
12. What is meant by 30 volume hydrogen peroxide? What percentage strength is equivalent to 30 volume hydrogen peroxide?
13. What are the main uses of hydrogen peroxide in a salon?
14. How would you dilute 60 volume hydrogen peroxide to 20 volume?

TYPES OF HAIR COLOURING

Hair colourings are classified into the following groups:

- **Natural vegetable dyes**, which include henna, walnut and camomile.

- **Metallic dyes,** such as sulphide dyes, which are used only in home hairdressing but may cause problems for the hairdresser.
- **Synthetic dyes,** which may be subdivided into
  - (a) temporary colours, mostly azo dyes
  - (b) semi-permanent colours or nitro dyes
  - (c) permanent oxidation dyes or para dyes.

VEGETABLE DYES

Vegetable dyes have a very limited range of colour, but are unlikely to cause dermatitis and are non-toxic.

Camomile

Camomile (or chamomile) is prepared from the dried flowers of the camomile plant, the active ingredient being **apigenin**. The dye coats the hair shaft giving a yellow cast, the molecules being too large to enter the cortex. Camomile is used as a rinse after shampooing or is added to hair lightening and brightening shampoos for use on blonde or light brown hair.

Walnut

Walnut produces a brown colour. The juice of unripe walnut shells is used to give a permanent colour. Some modern colour shampoos contain walnut to deepen the colour of dark brown hair.

Henna

Henna is obtained from the dried leaves of the Egyptian privet Lawsonia Alba and the active ingredient is **lawsone**. It gives a permanent colour by penetrating the hair shaft to produce red shades, which may be emphasized by the addition of acetic acid or made slightly browner by the addition of borax (alkaline). If the leaves are collected before fully mature the product is known as **Green Henna**, and this gives a more delicate shade of red than normal henna. Indigo, from the plant of that name, used to be mixed with henna to produce **Persian Henna** or **Henna Reng**, which dyed hair a magnificent blue-black colour. Modern colour shampoos may contain henna to give auburn highlights to brown and chestnut hair. It is also used as a dye on black hair and gives an attractive red cast, particularly in bright sunlight.

METALLIC DYES

Inorganic salts are used in **hair colour restorers**. Lead salts or silver salts applied to the hair gradually darken by the action of hydrogen sulphide in the air, and so 'restore' hair colour. The effect may be increased by the addition of sodium thiosulphate to the salts.

In **two-application dyes**, or **sulphide dyes**, the hair is first treated with sodium sulphide solution and then with the solution of a metallic salt such as lead acetate, silver nitrate or copper sulphate. Double decomposition takes place and a metal sulphide is deposited both in the cortex and on the surface of the hair.

For example:

sodium sulphide + copper sulphate → sodium sulphate + copper sulphide
(black)

Disadvantages of metallic dyes

Metallic dyes have many disadvantages.

- Some, such as lead and copper salts, are poisonous.
- They give a dull appearance to the hair.
- Strong sodium sulphide is a depilatory (hair remover).
- Perming or bleaching cannot be carried out on hair previously treated with metallic salts. Copper and iron salts may act as catalysts, causing vigorous decomposition of hydrogen peroxide (used in bleaches and in neutralizer during perming) resulting in hair breakage.

Compound henna

Compound henna consists of a mixture of henna and silver, copper or lead salts. A typical formula is:

henna	72 g
pyrogallic acid	12 g
copper sulphate	8 g
burnt sienna	8 g

The ingredients are mixed to a paste with water at about 70°C before use. The presence of metallic dyes make these preparations poisonous, and it is also difficult to perm the hair afterwards.

SYNTHETIC ORGANIC DYES

These form the most modern and widely used group of dyes. Some are based on coal tar dyes or aniline dyes.

Temporary dyes

Temporary dyes have molecules which are normally too big to enter the cortex unless the hair is very porous. They usually just coat the outside of the hair shaft. Exposure to the sun may cause fading of temporary colour and some colour is lost gradually by brushing. The dyes are unlikely to cause allergic reaction and a skin test is not required before use. Temporary dyes are applied in various forms but all wash out at the first shampoo.

Colour rinses

Colour rinses are used after shampooing and are allowed to dry on the hair. They may contain cationic dyes such as methylene blue and methyl violet, which cling to the acid groups of the hair. More often they are formulated with anionic (acidic) azo dyes such as para-hydroxyazobenzene (yellow) and phenylazonaphthol (red). Organic acids such as citric or tartaric acids are added to give a pH of 4.

Coloured setting lotions

Coloured setting lotions contain acid azo dyes added to a plastic film former, which is dissolved in alcohol and water. A coloured plastic film is left on the hair after drying. Coloured setting aids may also be formulated as mousses and gels (see Chapter 13).

Colour sprays

Colour sprays also contain azo dyes together with plastic resin dissolved in alcohol. The colour is sprayed on to the hair after dressing out. Finely powdered aluminium may be added to some lacquers to give a silver lustre.

Colour shampoos

Colour shampoos may contain synthetic azo dyes added to the detergent along with organic acids such as citric acid or lactic acid to give a pH value of about 5. The shampoos do not produce a marked change in hair colour but brighten faded hair and add highlights.

Crayons, paints, mousses and gels

Coloured crayons, paints, mousses and gels containing temporary colours (azo dyes) may be applied after the hair has been styled and dried to give colour exactly where required.

Semi-permanent dyes

Semi-permanent dyes consist of mixtures of nitro dyes, which give red and yellow colours, and anthraquinones, which give blue colours, for example:

> dinitro-amino-phenol (picramic acid) (red)
> nitro-phenylenediamine (yellow)
> tetra-amino-anthraquinone (blue)

Varous mixtures of these three colours produce a wide range of shades. The dyes are already in a coloured form and the molecules are small enough to enter the cortex. This takes some time but does not involve a chemical reaction. The dye mixture is made alkaline to pH 8 to aid penetration into the cortex and quarternary ammonium compounds are added to ensure an even distribution of colour. During processing the head may be covered with a plastic cap and heat applied from a steamer or infra-red heater to speed penetration.

In the hair shaft, the dye molecules partly join in the hydrogen bonds. Each time the hair is washed, water replaces some of the dye in the bonds, and the dye gradually washes out in six to eight shampoos. The dye washes out of bleached hair more easily because it is more porous.

In a brown dye consisting of a mixture of red, yellow and blue dyes, difficulties sometimes occur because the red and yellow dye molecules are smaller than those of the blue dye. Extra blue dye is often added during manufacture to ensure that sufficient enters the hair shaft to give a good colour. If the hair is very porous, for example immediately after a perm, too much blue may enter and upset the colour balance. Similarly the dyes do not wash out equally and a slight change of colour may occur each time the hair is shampooed. Brown semi-permanent dyes tend to be reddish or golden.

Quasi-permanent dyes

By themselves semi-permanent dyes are safe and no skin test is required before use. However, some semi-permanent dyes are mixed with permanent oxidation dyes and are then known as quasi-permanent dyes. The dye base has to be mixed with hydrogen peroxide immediately before use. This type of dye may cause an allergic reaction in some people and **a skin test** is required at least 24 hours before it is intended to apply the dye. (Skin tests are described in Chapter 10).

Removal of semi-permanent dyes

Unwanted semi-permanent dye on the hair can be removed by repeated shampooing or by use of a spirit soap as the dyes are more soluble in spirit than in water. Use four parts of soft soap dissolved in one part of industrial methylated spirit.

Permanent oxidation dyes

The earliest oxidation dyes were para-phenylenediamine (diamino-benzene) which produced a black compound on oxidation, and para-toluenediamine (diamino-toluene) which produced a brown compound. The series of dyes thus became known as **para dyes**. A large number of other chemicals have now been added to the series to give a wider range of colours. These include:

> para-aminophenol (reddish brown)
> meta-dihydroxybenzene (grey)
> meta-phenylenediamine (brown)

Mixtures of these dyes are prepared as thick liquids or creams designed to be mixed with 20 volume hydrogen peroxide immediately before use. The following substances are added to the mixture of dyes during manufacture:

- ammonium hydroxide (producing a pH of about 9) to raise the cuticle scales and allow easy penetration of the dye molecules, and to catalyse the decomposition of the hydrogen peroxide, so releasing oxygen
- sodium sulphite (a reducing agent) to prevent premature oxidation of the dye
- conditioners such as lanolin and cetyl alcohol
- foaming agents such as triethanolamine soaps, to facilitate rinsing off the excess dye.

The final colour of the dye is reached only by oxidation, which takes

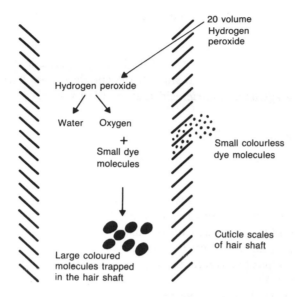

20 volume
Hydrogen
peroxide

Hydrogen peroxide

Water   Oxygen
+
Small dye
molecules

Small colourless
dye molecules

Large coloured
molecules trapped
in the hair shaft

Cuticle scales
of hair shaft

Fig. 15.10   Permanent colour

place inside the hair shaft. The small colourless dye molecules enter the cortex along with hydrogen peroxide. On oxidation, large coloured molecules are formed which become trapped in the hair shaft as they are too large to wash out (see Fig. 15.10). The dye thus produces a permanent colour, but the periodic dyeing of the new growth of hair is essential if the colour is to be maintained.

small colourless   oxygen from   large coloured molecules which
   dye molecules   +   hydrogen peroxide →   become trapped in the cortex

The oxidation reaction is slow and may take 10 to 30 minutes to complete, but the dye should not be mixed with hydrogen peroxide until required for use, as any large molecules formed would not then be able to enter the hair shaft. On the hair, oxidation may be speeded by heat from a steamer, an accelerator or infra-red heater.

Unless the hair is very dark, replacing 20 volume hydrogen peroxide by 30 volume strength enables bleaching and dyeing to take place at the same time, and the hair may be dyed lighter than the natural shade. Very dark or black hair may need pre-lightening with hydrogen peroxide before colouring in order to obtain a satisfactory lighter shade.

Oxidation dyes are easy to use and give a good range of natural looking colours. Some fading may take place if the hair is subjected to strong sunlight, but under normal conditions the colour is maintained well.

There is no difficulty if hair is permed later, though there may be a slight loss of colour.

After the dye has been rinsed from the hair, anti-oxidant and acid rinses may be used to stop further action of the hydrogen peroxide, to neutralize any alkali on the hair and to smooth the cuticle scales. Ascorbic acid (a reducing agent) and citric acid may be used for this purpose.

Contra-indications to the use of para dyes

Oxidation dyes should not be applied to the hair if any of the following conditions apply:

- There are cuts or abrasions on the scalp.
- There are any signs of disease of the scalp or hair.
- Metallic salts are present on the hair.
- The hair itself is in very poor condition.
- There is a positive reaction to a skin test (see details of skin tests in Chapter 10).
- The hair has just been permed.

Removal of permanent dyes (strippers)

If, due to a mistake, it is necessary to remove a permanent oxidation dye from the hair, **reduction** (the reverse of oxidation) must take place. Strong reducing agents such as sodium formaldehyde sulphoxylate or sodium bisulphate are required. Overuse of these reducing agents may lead to serious breakdown of cystine linkages in the hair.

Safety notes

- Do not shampoo the hair before tinting because shampooing makes the skin more sensitive.
- Always wear protective gloves when applying para dyes, not only to avoid staining the skin but also to prevent dye dermatitis.
- Never use hair dyes on the eyebrows or lashes. Certain chemicals used in hair dyes are not permitted in colours intended to be used in the more sensitive area around the eyes.
- Never allow dyes to enter a cut.
- Always give a skin test before applying a para dye.
- Use barrier cream to protect the client's skin at the hair line and over the ears.

SELF TESTING

1. Name three types of vegetable dyes and state the colour each will produce.
2. What is (a) apigenin (b) lawsone (c) compound henna?
3. Why is it important to detect the presence of metallic salts on the hair?
4. What is meant by (a) hair colour restorer (b) a depilatory?
5. What is the effect on the hair of (a) temporary dyes (b) semi-permanent dyes (c) permanent dyes?
6. What type of colour is produced by (a) para dyes (b) azo dyes (c) nitro dyes?
7. What is meant by a quasi-permanent dye? Is a skin test required for this type of dye?
8. What type of chemical reaction takes place during (a) permanent colouring (b) removal of a permanent dye from the hair?
9. For what types of dyes is a skin test required? What is the purpose of the test? How is the test carried out?
10. During manufacture, what chemical substances are added to the dye base of a permanent dye? For what purposes are they added?
11. How and where is the final colour produced during permanent tinting?
12. How may an unwanted semi-permanent dye be removed from the hair?

BLEACHING

The aim of bleaching is to decolourize hair pigments with as little damage to the hair as possible. Bleaching takes place by oxidation of the natural pigments in the hair.

Black and brown pigments are more easily oxidized than red and yellow pigments, so that the oxidation takes place in three stages:

- oxidation of black and brown pigments leaving red and yellow
- oxidation of red pigment leaving yellow
- oxidation of yellow pigment

The oxygen required for bleaching is usually obtained from the decomposition of hydrogen peroxide, ammonium hydroxide being added as a catalyst to speed the release of oxygen. A **catalyst** is a substance which speeds up a reaction but remains unchanged itself at the end of the reaction. Hydrogen peroxide, because it supplies oxygen for the reaction, is known as an **oxidizing agent**.

$$\text{Hydrogen peroxide} \longrightarrow \text{oxygen} + \text{water}$$

Newly formed oxygen or **nascent** (new-born) **oxygen** is a powerful bleaching agent unlike ordinary atmospheric oxygen. The oxidation process of bleaching is represented by the following equation:

$$\begin{array}{ccc}
\text{Melanin} & \text{nascent oxygen} & \text{oxy-melanin} \\
\text{(coloured)} \ + & \text{(from hydrogen peroxide)} \longrightarrow & \text{(colourless)}
\end{array}$$

PROCEDURE BEFORE BLEACHING

Examine hair and scalp

Look for cuts, abrasions or any sign of disease on the scalp or hair. Do not bleach if these are present.

Consult client

Consult the client about any previous home and salon treatments. Refer to the client's record card if available.

Check condition

Test the hair if you think it may have low tensile strength and high porosity. Do not bleach hair which is in poor condition. A test cutting of hair taken from an inconspicuous area of the client's head may be pre-tested with bleach to assess the result.

Test for incompatibility

Carry out an incompatibility test (see Chapter 10) if you suspect the client has used metallic dye or compound henna on the hair previously.

COMPOSITION OF BLEACHES

Bleaching preparations contain two parts which are mixed immediately before use. Bleach must not be left standing after mixing or oxygen will be lost and the bleach will not be effective.

Oxidizing agent

An oxidizing agent, usually hydrogen peroxide but occasionally magnesium peroxide, is used to provide nascent oxygen for bleaching.

Alkali

An alkaline substance, usually ammonium hydroxide solution (or solid ammonium carbonate in paste bleaches) to give a pH of 8−9.5. The alkali has no bleaching power itself.

Functions of the alkali

- to neutralize the acid stabilizer in the peroxide
- to act as a wetting agent and cause the hair to swell to allow greater penetration of the peroxide into the hair shaft
- to act as a catalyst to speed the release oxygen from the peroxide.

Safety notes

- Do not shampoo the hair before bleaching as this increases skin sensitivity.
- Strong hydrogen peroxide, at strengths over 30 volume (9 per cent), can burn the skin.
- Protect the client's hair line and the tops of the ears with barrier cream before a full head bleach.
- Always wear protective gloves when applying bleach.
- Do not overlap when retouching bleach or breakage may occur.
- Wear a face mask when mixing powder bleaches.

TYPES OF BLEACHES

Liquid bleach

Simple liquid bleach contains 20 volume (6 per cent) hydrogen peroxide which is mixed immediately before use with ammonium hydroxide of pH 8.5 thickened with a little soapless shampoo. It is capable only of limited lightening of hair colour so is used to revive blonde hair which has darkened with age or to give highlights to light brown hair.

Cream bleaches

Cream bleaches consists of an alkaline cream or emulsion with a pH of about 9 with added cetrimide as a conditioner. This is mixed with 20 volume (6 per cent) hydrogen peroxide immediately before use. The thick emulsion holds the hydrogen peroxide in close contact with the hair during bleaching. Boosters of potassium persulphate or ammonium persulphate may be added at the same time as the peroxide to provide more oxygen and so increase bleaching power.

Oil bleaches

Oil bleaches contain sulphonated caster oil (Turkey red oil) as a thickener with an alkali to give a pH of 9. This is mixed with 20 volume (6 per cent) hydrogen peroxide just before use. Oil bleaches give a golden blonde shade and do not bleach as completely as cream or paste bleaches.

Powder or paste bleaches

Powder or paste bleaches consist of a mixture of two white powders, magnesium carbonate forming the bulk of the powder and ammonium carbonate as the alkali to give a pH of 8.5. (Magnesium carbonate is sometimes referred to as white henna but has no connection with the vegetable dye of red henna). Immediately before use, the powders are mixed to a smooth paste with 6–9 per cent hydrogen peroxide for general bleaching or 9–12 per cent hydrogen peroxide for bleached streaks or tips. Because the hydrogen peroxide is not diluted by any other liquid, paste bleaches are more likely to cause hair damage than other types of bleach, and the hair may be left rough and porous. Care must be taken not to inhale the powders when mixing the bleach. The use of a **face mask** is advised.

Gel bleaches

Gel bleaches rely on the formation of a thick gel when hydrogen peroxide is added. Many modern bleaches are of this type. The bleach base consists of three ingredients:

- **ammonium hydroxide** to give a pH of 9–9.5, which makes the hair swell and speeds the release of oxygen from the hydrogen peroxide
- a cationic **wetting agent**, e.g. cetrimide
- a **gelling agent** or thickener, usually a non-ionic detergent such as

lauryl diethanolamide which thickens and increases in bulk when 6 per cent hydrogen peroxide is added immediately before use.

To increase the amount of available oxygen, **boosters** of potassium persulphate or ammonium persulphate may be added at the same time as the peroxide. The gelling agent is sometimes added to the booster instead of to the alkali. Carbopol (a carboxyl vinyl polymer) is used for this purpose as it gels on contact with the alkali.

TREATMENTS AFTER BLEACHING

The bleach must be rinsed out of the hair with tepid water as soon as the correct amount of lightening has been achieved or the hair may quickly over bleach. Unless the bleach is to be followed by a toner, an anti-oxidant rinse is also advisable immediately after bleaching.

Anti-oxidant rinse

This type of rinse with a pH of 4 contains anti-oxidants, acids and conditioners.

- Anti-oxidants are mild reducing agents, such as ascorbic acid, which stop any further oxidation inside the hair shaft.
- Acids, such as citric acid, neutralize any alkali left on the hair, smooth the cuticle scales and return the hair to its normal acid state. They also prevent the loss from the hair of water-soluble products produced from keratin during bleaching.
- Conditioners of the cetrimide type, which are substantive to hair, are used because they are attracted electrostatically to the increased number of negatively charged acid groups present in hair after bleaching.

Use of toners

Light brown or blonde hair will usually lighten satisfactorily without further treatment but darker hair may be left slightly yellow after bleaching. To mask unwanted yellow or to add colour to lightened hair, pastel toners can be used after bleaching. These may be weak forms of temporary, semi-permanent or permanent dyes designed to give delicate colours such as beige, silver or rose.

Weak solutions of cationic temporary dyes such as methylene blue or methyl violet may be used to disguise yellowness after bleaching or to produce a platinum blonde. They are substantive to hair and cling electrostatically to the acid groups of the hair. Care must be taken with the strength of solution as too much blue may give the hair a green cast (yellow + blue = green). Temporary acidic azo dyes may also be used.

Most modern toners are mixtures of semi-permanent dyes to give delicate pastel shades and usually include a little violet dye to counteract yellowness after bleaching.

If permanent dyes are to be used after bleaching, a skin sensitivity test must be given at least 24 hours before the proposed application of dye. The dye should be mixed with 10 volume hydrogen peroxide only. Higher strength peroxide would cause hair damage.

HAIR DAMAGE DURING BLEACHING

Bleaching is, in general, more damaging to hair than perming or tinting, especially if bleaching dark hair to blonde. A mild bleach taking a longer time does less damage than a strong bleach used for a shorter time. There are three main areas of damage by bleaching.

Permanent loss of disulphide bonds

Permanent loss of disulphide bonds between the polypeptide chains in keratin is caused by oxidation of cystine to cysteic acid. This reduces the tensile strength of the hair. When the hair is wet, water entering the narrow spaces between the chains by capillary rise may force the chains apart, causing the hair to swell and become water logged. It is then difficult to dry out but when dry becomes straw-like. Some oxidation products of keratin are soluble and may be washed out of the hair leading to further weakening. Loss of bonds may make it inadvisable to perm hair after bleaching.

Breakage of polypeptide chains

Breakage of polypeptide chains is caused by over-bleaching, the use of hydrogen peroxide which is too strong, or solutions which are too alkaline, causing breakage of the hair shaft.

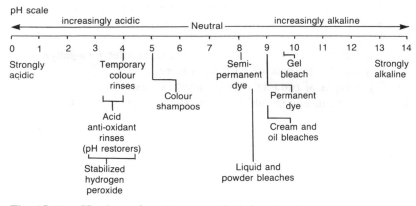

Fig. 15.11 pH values of products used in hair colouring

Cuticle damage

Structural damage to the cuticle may be caused, especially during retouching if overlapping occurs. The scales may be roughened or broken off, leading to increased porosity. Further damage may occur later unless the hair is treated gently during brushing and combing.

pH VAI UES

The pH values of products used in hair colouring are shown in Fig. 15.11.

SELF TESTING

1. What is the aim of bleaching?
2. Describe the stages which take place during bleaching of dark hair.
3. What is meant by a catalyst?
4. What is nascent oxygen and how does it differ from the oxygen of the air?
5. What type of chemical reaction takes place during bleaching?
6. What is the purpose of (a) hydrogen peroxide (b) ammonium hydroxide in bleaches?
7. What is meant by a bleach booster? Give an example of a substance used as a booster.

8. Why should a bleach not be left standing after mixing?
9. What are the main ingredients of a paste bleach?
10. What is the effect of over-bleaching?
11. What type of rinse is considered beneficial after bleaching?
12. What is the purpose of a bleach toner?
13. What types of product may be used as toners?
14. What precautions should be taken when using bleaches and toners?

PART 5
HAIRDRESSING FOR AFRO CLIENTS

16

AFRO HAIRDRESSING

The distinctive characteristics of Afro hair require special hairdressing techniques, which are in some respects quite different from those used on European hair. The actual chemical structure of hair keratin is, however, the same in both cases. The structure of polypeptide chains with salt linkages, cystine linkages and hydrogen bonds is identical. The most obvious difference is in the tightness of the curl in Afro hair. This may be due to follicle shape, but also to uneven keratinization leading to the formation of an ortho cortex and para cortex. This dual cortex can be detected in very curly hair by certain staining techniques followed by microscopic examination of cross-sections of hairs (see Fig. 16.1). The ortho cortex has a less dense structure than the para cortex and always lies on the outside of the wave (refer back to Fig. 14.2).

AFRO HAIR

Afro hair has various characteristics, as follows.

- Tightness of **curl** may disguise the actual length of Afro hair, which is often quite long when straightened.
- The **direction** of hair growth varies throughout the head, and the hair does not fall into a regular wave pattern or natural partings.
- Afro hair has intense black **pigmentation**.
- **Texture** (hair diameter) varies along the hair shaft, creating some narrow segments where the hair is weaker and more easily broken. As in European hair, Afro hair can be divided according to texture into fine, medium and coarse hair. Fine Afro hair tends to be woolly and is soft and spongy. The majority of people have medium textured hair which lies between fine and coarse. Coarse hair tends to be

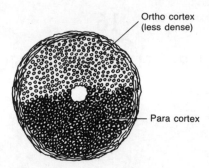

Fig. 16.1 Section of ortho cortex and para cortex

difficult to manage, resistant to chemical treatment and rather stiff
or hard to the touch.
- **Porosity** also varies along the hair shaft leading to uneven uptake of
  chemicals and possible chemical damage at weaker points.
- Afro hair tends to be **dry** and needs frequent oil treatments both for
  the hair and skin of the scalp. Dryness is often increased by frequent
  straightening by heat or by chemical treatment.

AFRO SKIN

Afro skin has characteristics which enable it to withstand radiation from
the sun of both heat and ultra-violet rays.

Pigmentation

Pigmentation is important as the melanin in the skin absorbs ultra-violet
rays which otherwise causes skin damage. All types of skin have
approximately the same number of **melanocytes** (cells in the germinating
layer of the epidermis which produces granules of the pigment melanin),
but dark skins produce more melanin granules and the size of the granules
is greater than in white skin. Again in dark skins the melanin is present
in the outer horny layer of the skin but in white skin the melanin is
destroyed by enzyme action before it reaches the horny layer. The
increased amount of pigment means that dark skins absorb more radiant
heat than white skins. The pigment in dark skins also sometimes hides
defects of the skin and affects the colour produced by massage or heat
treatment. Hyperaemia (increase of the blood supply to the skin)
produces erythema (redness) in a white skin but a purple colour in dark
skin.

Sweat glands

The number and size of sweat glands is greater in dark than in white skins and the pores are more noticeable. More sweat is secreted and as evaporation of sweat cools the skin, this compensates for the increased absorption of radiant heat.

Sebaceous glands

Sebaceous glands in the skin are more numerous and larger than in white skin, with many opening on to the skin itself rather than into the hair follicles. Extra sebum production cuts down the amount of ultra-violet light entering the skin. Small cysts of sebum sometimes develop in the follicles but are obvious only to the touch.

Epidermis

The horny layer of the epidermis is thick and tough, and dark skin sheds the outer scales readily sometimes producing a grey cast on the skin.

Keloids

When Afro skin is damaged, keloids sometimes form as the skin heals. These consist of permanent scar tissue which becomes raised above the surface of the skin. Great care should therefore be taken not to damage Afro skin.

FEATURES OF THE HEAD

Hair styling always involves a study of the main features of the client's head including facial features.

The typical bone structure of the Afro skull includes

- a deep forehead
- high cheek bones
- flat nasal bones
- a prominent jaw.

The high cheek bones and the prominence of the jaw lend good support to the skin. Bone support, coupled with melanin which protects the skin from sun damage, results in delayed ageing of black skin until about the age of 60 years. Typical facial features include the broadness of the nose and the fullness of the lips.

SELF TESTING

1. In what ways does typical Afro hair differ from European hair?
2. Does the chemical structure of Afro hair differ from that of European hair?
3. What are the main characteristics of (a) fine Afro hair (b) coarse Afro hair?
4. What are the main characteristics of Afro skin?
5. What is meant by a keloid?
6. Why does Afro skin age less quickly than European skin?
7. What typical features of the head and face have to be taken into consideration when deciding on a style for Afro hair?

GENERAL CARE OF AFRO HAIR

The tightness of the curl and the uneven texture of Afro hair means that breakage of the hair shaft often occurs during normal grooming. Combing, if not carried out with care using a **wide toothed comb** or Afro comb, can cause breakages even in virgin hair (hair which is untreated chemically). Jagged broken-off ends also tend to cause matting or tangling of adjacent hairs leading to further difficulties when combing. Although Afro hair grows at the same rate as European hair (1.25 cm per month) constant breakage may make the growth rate seem slower.

Hot combing or pressing to straighten extra tight curls makes the hair easier to manage and to groom, but if applied too frequently results in loss of oils from the surface of the hair. This in turn leads to loss of moisture from the hair shaft which becomes dry and brittle with the possibility of further breakage. Dry, brittle hair may also result from the too frequent use of chemicals in carrying out curly perms or straightening.

To keep natural Afro hair in good condition:

- Brush and comb the hair carefully and gently. Application of a moisturizing spray containing oils or glycerol (glycerine) makes the hair easier to comb and decreases the risk of hair breakage.
- Use conditioning shampoos containing protein hydrolysates, which make the hair smoother by providing a protective coat to the hair shaft.
- Avoid frequent use of chemical or heat treatments.

- Condition the hair frequently with oil based or protein based conditioners.
- Cut the hair every few weeks to remove split ends and prevent tangling.

CONDITIONERS AND CONDITIONING TREATMENTS

The dryness of Afro hair makes conditioning particularly important.

Moisturizing

Steaming is useful to restore moisture to the hair and to increase elasticity especially after frequent heat treatments. **Oil based conditioners** act as moisturizers by preventing loss of moisture from the hair shaft, and make the hair easier to comb. **Protein hydrolysates** reduce tangling and also reduce the porosity of the hair. **Glycerol and propylene glycol** are often used in conditioners for Afro hair as a humectant to attract moisture to the hair shaft. **Cream rinses** (cetrimide rinses) used after shampooing are suitable for virgin Afro hair.

Deep conditioning

Deep conditioning is essential for at least two weeks before relaxing by caustic alkalis. Traditionally this was by **hot oil treatments** using either olive oil or mineral oils, assisted by heat from hot towels or from a steamer. More modern deep conditioners contain **cationic** conditioners, **humectants** such as glycerol, and **protein hydrolysates** as well as mineral oils, in a thick cream emulsion. These deep conditioners should be applied to the hair, covered by a plastic cap and heated under a hood dryer for 20 minutes before being rinsed off. Similar deep conditioners are required after relaxing to counteract the degreasing effect of the strong alkali. Conditioners for use after a curly perm may contain protein hydrolysates or cationic conditioners and propylene glycol as a humectant.

SHAMPOOS

Pre-perm shampoos

Pre-perm shampoos should be mild (not too degreasing) with a pH of 7 and may contain protein hydrolysates to even out the porosity of the hair. They should be used with a minimum of massage to avoid total removal of oils from the skin of the scalp, which would leave the skin more sensitive to chemical irritation.

Neutralizing shampoos

Neutralizing shampoos are designed to chemically neutralize any alkali left on the hair after use of caustic alkali relaxers and so stop further action. They should be used for no other purpose. The shampoos contain citric acid to produce a pH of 4–5, and the detergent base is usually ammonium lauryl sulphate with protein hydrolysates as conditioners. A chemical indicator (phenolphthalein) may be included in the shampoo to show, by colour change in the lather, the presence of alkali remaining in the hair. This indicator is pink in alkaline solution but colourless in acid solution.

Conditioning shampoos

Conditioning shampoos for general use on chemically treated hair contain protein hydrolysate conditioners in an ammonium lauryl sulphate shampoo base, with lactic acid or citric acid added to produce a pH of 6.

PLAITING

Various forms of plaiting such as cane row or corn row and French braiding are traditional in Afro hairdressing. An **oily pomade** containing a mixture of lanolin, mineral oils and petroleum jelly is applied to the hair to prevent damage while the hair is being combed out and plaited in the desired style. The tension applied to the hair by repeated plaiting may lead to traction alopecia (refer back to Fig. 8.9).

WET SETTING

Wet setting (roller setting) is not very satisfactory on virgin Afro hair as stretching is limited and the hair soon reverts to its natural tightly curled state. Roller setting may, however, be carried out after relaxing. Plastic resin setting lotions or styling gels are used as setting aids (see Chapter 13). Dressing creams, containing light mineral oils, lanolin products and humectants such as propylene glycol, may be applied to provide gloss and act as moisturizers.

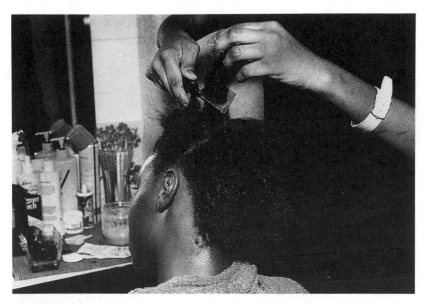

Fig. 16.2 Hot pressing

THERMAL STRAIGHTENING OR HOT PRESSING

Temporary straightening of hair by heat can be carried out by hair pressing with heated combs (see Fig. 16.2), the use of curling tongs, or by flat irons (that is by pressing the hair between two flat heated surfaces). The process is a physical one involving the rearrangement of hydrogen bonds by heating and stretching the hair as in the temporary heat setting (dry setting) of European hair, and lasts only until the hair is next shampooed.

There are two types of hair pressing by heated combs

- **soft pressing** in which the hair over the whole head is pressed once only with a heated metal comb
- **hard pressing** is a second pressing over the soft press again using a heated metal comb.

PROCEDURE FOR HOT PRESSING

Shampoo and dry hair

The hair is first shampooed, rinsed and then dried using either a hood or blow dryer. This ensures that the hair shaft contains the maximum amount of water before pressing begins. Shampooing allows more water to enter the hair shaft than if the hair is just wetted because the shampoo acts as a wetting agent by lowering surface tension.

Apply pressing cream or oil

Pressing cream or oil is applied evenly but sparingly over the hair. The cream may be in the form of (a) a pomade containing mineral oils, lanolin, petroleum jelly and petroleum waxes or (b) a silicone oil emulsion which forms a waterproof layer to protect the hair from loss of set, by preventing absorption of moisture when processing is completed. Pressing oils act as a protective layer between the comb and hair, and prevent damage by lubricating the hair to reduce drag on the comb. They also help to conduct the heat from the comb to the hair.

Test temperature of heated comb

The temperature of the heated pressing comb should be tested on a piece of tissue paper. If scorching occurs, the comb must be allowed to cool before being applied to the hair.

Exert pressure with comb

The back of the hot comb is used to exert pressure on the hair. Greater pressure is required if the hair is coarse, and lighter pressure on fine woolly hair. Hard pressing is carried out if the soft press produces insufficient straightening.

Condition hair

To improve hair condition, a little pressing oil should be brushed through the hair on completion of pressing.

HAIR DAMAGE DURING HOT PRESSING

Hair breakage

Heating and stretching the hair may cause hair breakage.

Loss of elasticity

The cortex of the hair may lose moisture leading to loss of elasticity, and to dry brittle hair which is liable to breakage during normal brushing and combing.

Cuticle damage

The cuticle may be damaged by frequent hot pressing and portions may break away.

Traction alopecia

Tension on the hair may lead to traction alopecia, particularly at the front hairline if hot pressing is used frequently.

Scalp burns

Scalp burns may occur unless great care is taken. Burning of both the hair and scalp may result if the comb is too hot.

SELF TESTING

1. Why may lack of care in normal grooming of Afro hair cause hair breakage?
2. What is the effect of loss of oils from the hair by frequent straightening using hot pressing?
3. Why should natural Afro hair be cut every few weeks?
4. Name a chemical often used as a humectant in conditioners for Afro hair.
5. What are the ingredients of a modern deep conditioner? When is this type of conditioner used?
6. What is the purpose of a neutralizing shampoo? What are the main ingredients of the shampoo?
7. What is meant by traction alopecia? How may it be caused?
8. What is meant by soft and hard pressing? What damage to the hair and scalp may be caused by hot pressing?

CURLY PERM

The object of a curly perm or rearrangement of curl for Afro hair is to lessen the amount of curl in natural tightly curled Afro hair, resulting in a much looser type of curl. The perming process is based on chemical reduction by the application of ammonium thioglycollate in two stages, followed by neutralizing (chemical oxidation) and conditioning. Perming may be carried out on virgin Afro hair or as a root retouch on previously permed Afro hair.

PROCEDURE BEFORE PERMING

Examine the hair for condition (elasticity, tensile strength and porosity), and assess previous treatment from both heat and chemical processing.

- A perm cannot be carried out on previously chemically **relaxed hair** as there are insufficient disulphide bonds left in relaxed hair to produce a satisfactory perm. Relaxed hair is also usually very dry and easily broken.
- If a regrowth perm is to be carried out, care must be taken not to overlap **previously permed** areas as hair breakage may occur. The growth areas can best be defined by applying products containing protein hydrolysates (similar to pre-perm fillers) to release the curl. Shampooing is used for this purpose when perming European hair, but for Afro hair shampooing before perming is not normally recommended.
- If the hair is in **poor condition** due to previous heat or chemical treatments several deep conditioning treatments are advisable before attempting a curly perm.
- If **porosity** is uneven, cream or liquid protein hydrolysate fillers may be massaged into the porous areas and the product left in the hair during perming. The product should be used according to the manufacturer's instructions.
- If you are unsure about the success of the perm for any reason, a series of **test curls** should be made at various sites using the same perm and neutralizing products as in the intended perm. The results can then be assessed.
- If the hair is coated with oils a mild protein-based shampoo may be used but otherwise **no shampoo** should be given before perming. Massage should be gentle and the water tepid to avoid the removal of too much oil from the scalp.

- Before perming, a protective layer of **barrier cream** or vaseline should be applied round the client's hair line and the tops of the ears to prevent skin damage.
- To **avoid dermatitis** the hairdresser should always wear protective gloves during perming.

STAGES IN PERMING

First stage of perming

The hair is first straightened by use of an ammonium thioglycollate **straightener** or **rearranger**. Ingredients in the straightener are as follows:

- A **thick cream** (an emulsion of mineral oils and water) or a carbopol gel to hold the product in place on the hair and help to weigh down and straighten the curl during processing.
- A reducing agent of **10–12 per cent ammonium thioglycollate** to break down some of the disulphide bonds of hair keratin. The product is available in several different strengths depending on the type, texture and previous treatment of the hair.
- **Ammonium hydroxide** (pH 9.5) to aid penetration of the reducing agent into the hair.
- **Hydrolysed protein** as a conditioner.

The product is designed to be left on the hair for between 20 and 30 minutes. A plastic cap may be used over the hair to retain body heat and so speed processing. The chemical process is shown in Fig. 16.3.

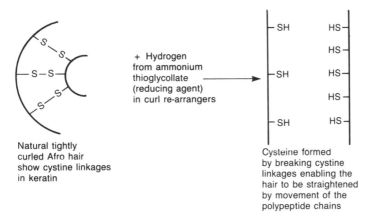

Natural tightly curled Afro hair show cystine linkages in keratin

+ Hydrogen from ammonium thioglycollate (reducing agent) in curl re-arrangers

Cysteine formed by breaking cystine linkages enabling the hair to be straightened by movement of the polypeptide chains

Fig. 16.3 First stage of a curly perm

As soon as the hair is straight, smooth and pliable, the first stage of processing is complete. The hair must then be rinsed with tepid water for about 5 minutes and blotted dry with a towel.

Second stage of perming

A **curl booster** or **charger** containing a weaker solution of ammonium thioglycollate is applied to break more disulphide bonds, while the hair is moulded to the desired shape by winding on to large curlers according to the size of curl required. Some of the disulphide bonds have already been broken in the first stage of processing so the hair is in a delicate condition. No tension must be applied while winding the hair on to curlers or breakages may occur. Processing using a plastic cap is continued until on partly unwinding curlers from several different parts of the head (curl tests), the desired wave pattern is produced. All the perm lotion is then rinsed from the hair without removing the curlers. The chemical action and moulding are shown in Fig. 16.4.

Neutralizing

With the curlers still in place, neutralizer is applied to rebuild the disulphide bonds again to hold the hair in its new less tightly curled shape. The neutralizer may contain either hydrogen peroxide or sodium bromate as an oxidizing agent to re-form the bonds. Oxygen from the oxidizing

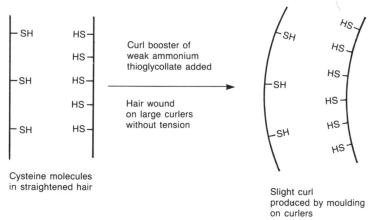

Fig. 16.4 Second stage of a curly perm

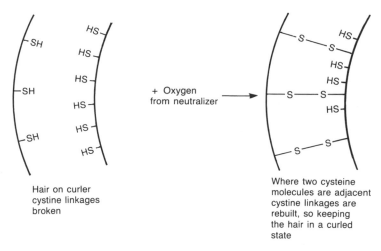

Hair on curler
cystine linkages
broken

+ Oxygen
from neutralizer

Where two cysteine
molecules are adjacent
cystine linkages are
rebuilt, so keeping
the hair in a curled
state

Fig. 16.5 Neutralizing a curly perm

agent removes hydrogen from the cysteine molecules and new cystine linkages are built. The chemical oxidation process during neutralizing is illustrated in Fig. 16.5. When neutralizing is complete the neutralizer is rinsed off and the curlers removed.

TREATMENTS AFTER PERMING

It is important to condition the hair immediately the neutralizer has been rinsed off the hair, because the double thioglycollate treatment leaves the hair with a rough and porous cuticle. The total package for a curly perm often includes a suitable **conditioner** as well as the perm lotions and the neutralizer. The conditioners may contain either quaternary ammonium compounds or protein hydrolysates at an acid pH of about 4 to chemically neutralize any alkali left on the hair, reduce swelling of the hair shaft and smooth the cuticle.

Alternative conditioners include:

- a **moisturizing spray** from a pressurized aerosol container to saturate the hair with a fine mist of humectant usually either propylene glycol or glycerol (glycerine), together with a conditioner of protein hydrolysates
- an **oil-based curl activator** containing mineral oils designed to replace sebum lost during processing and impart sheen to the hair, and a humectant usually glycerol to act as a moisturizer.

After dressing out, a hair spray containing silicones and lanolin will add shine and reduce the stickiness of the glycerol based conditioners.

Safety notes

- Keep the perm lotion off the skin as it may cause irritation.
- Take care not to over-process during perming as hair breakage may take place especially if overlapping occurs in a retouch perm. Check the progress of the perm according to the manufacturer's recommendations.
- Do not over-neutralize as the oxidizing agent may bleach natural colour and also result in fewer disulphide bonds being reformed as cystine may be oxidized to cysteic acid which does not form cross linkages.

CHEMICAL STRAIGHTENING OR RELAXING

Relaxing tightly curled hair or hair straightening is usually carried out using 1–4.5 per cent sodium hydroxide (sometimes known as **lye**) in a thick cream emulsion containing up to about 40 per cent of fatty material. Sodium hydroxide is a caustic alkali and has a pH of 13–14. If used incorrectly it will burn the skin and act as a depilatory by destroying hair.

'**No lye**' relaxers are available and consist of two parts: a **relaxer cream** containing calcium hydroxide, light mineral oils, paraffin jelly and non-ionic emulsifying waxes, and a **liquid activator** of guanidine carbonate in water which is added to the relaxer cream immediately before use. Guanidine hydroxide, an alkaline relaxing agent, is formed by chemical reaction and is less irritant than sodium hydroxide as the pH is lower (pH 10–12).

Calcium hydroxide + guanidine carbonate
→ guanidine hydroxide + calcium carbonate
(alkaline relaxer)

During relaxing, disulphide bonds are broken by a chemical process called hydrolysis, which means breaking up a substance by the addition of the elements of water (see Fig. 16.6). The product is designed to be left on the hair for about 20 minutes but the manufacturer's instructions must be closely followed if damage is to be avoided. The chemical reaction results in the formation of lanthionine linkages in hair keratin. These are permanent linkages containing only one sulphur atom instead of the two sulphur atoms in a cystine linkage. When the straightening is

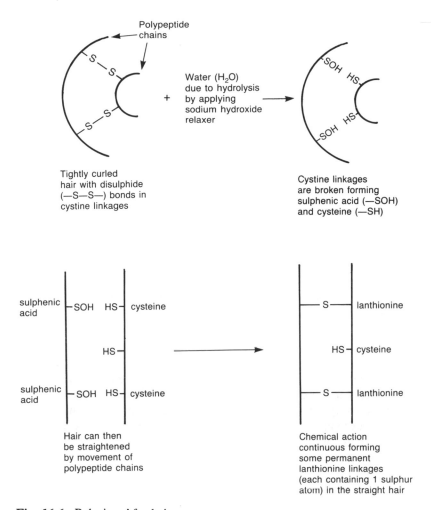

Fig. 16.6 Relaxing Afro hair

complete, the alkali must be washed out of the hair at a back-wash basin to prevent the alkali entering the client's eyes.

An acid based neutralizing shampoo (pH 4–5) must then be used to chemically neutralize any alkali left on the hair, stop futher action by the alkali, reduce the swelling of the hair shaft, and return the hair to its normal slightly acid state. (Note: The use of a neutralizing shampoo is a true chemical neutralization between an acid and an alkali, while neutralizing after thioglycollate perming is a chemical oxidation process.) The shampoo base is usually ammonium lauryl sulphate with the addition of citric acid. A chemical indicator, which will cause a colour change in the lather if any alkali is left on the hair, may be incorporated in the shampoo. Massage of the scalp during shampooing must be kept to a minimum because relaxing degreases the skin and leaves it sensitive.

PRECAUTIONS IN CHEMICAL STRAIGHTENING

- Hair straightening should not be attempted if the hair is in poor general condition or has had recent previous chemical treatment, e.g. perming.
- The scalp skin must be in good condition with no cuts or abrasions, otherwise severe irritation may occur.
- Several conditioning treatments are advisable in the weeks before straightening to ensure that the hair and scalp are well oiled. Oil slows down the relaxation process and reduces hair damage. The hair must not be shampooed immediately before straightening.
- The scalp skin including the hair line must be based thoroughly with vaseline or barrier cream before applying the straightener, unless the manufacturer's instructions indicate that the relaxer itself contains a basing oil. Failure to base can lead to chemical burns of the skin. Basing should always be carried out if the client's skin is known to be sensitive.
- To prevent serious burns, the caustic straightener must not come into contact with either the skin of the client or the skin of the hairdresser. Protective gloves are essential when applying hair straightener.
- Avoid over-processing as this can lead to the destruction of the hair. Always follow the manufacturer's instructions.
- Relaxed hair is delicate and must be treated gently after processing. Conditioning is essential as both the cuticle and internal bonds are damaged during processing.

TREATMENTS AFTER STRAIGHTENING

A deep conditioning treatment is essential after straightening, to repair damage to the hair and to return oil to the scalp. A cream emulsion with a high percentage of mineral oil, hydrolysed protein as a conditioner and glycerol as a humectant is suitable. The conditioner is best used along with heat treatment. A scalp grease containing mineral oils and lanolin may also be applied to the skin of the scalp to prevent dryness and possible flaking of the skin.

HAIR DAMAGE DURING CHEMICAL STRAIGHTENING

Chemical burns

Chemical burns may result if the caustic alkali relaxer comes into contact with the skin.

Swelling of hair shaft

Relaxer causes considerable swelling of the hair shaft.

Cuticle damage

Relaxer causes roughening of the cuticle scales. Some cuticle scales may break off.

Depilatory action

Relaxers have a high pH (10–14) and act as depilatories if left on the hair too long or if a strong relaxer is used on previously bleached or tinted hair. Strong alkalis (above pH 9.5) can destroy all the chemical bonds of keratin and cause complete disintegration and destruction of the hair.

Hair cannot be permed

Many cystine linkages (containing disulphide bonds) are replaced by lanthionine linkages (containing single sulphur atoms) during relaxing. Cystine linkages are essential in perming. Relaxed hair cannot be permed.

WARNING

- **Neutralizers** for use after a thioglycollate curly perm contain **oxidizing agents**.
- **Neutralizing shampoos** contain acids to **chemically neutralize** alkali left in the hair after use of relaxers.
- **Neutralizers and neutralizing shampoos are not interchangeable**.
- **Neutralizers (oxidizers)** intended for use after a thioglycollate curly perm must **never** be used to replace a neutralizing shampoo after relaxing Afro hair.

- **Neutralizing shampoos** intended for use after relaxers must **never** be used as neutralizers (oxidizers) for curly perms.

pH VALUES

The pH values of products used in curly perms and relaxing are shown in Fig. 16.7.

COLOURING

The types of colouring available for Afro hair are the same as for European hair (see Chapter 15).

Permanent dyes (para dyes)

Virgin Afro hair may be treated in the same way as European hair, though pre-lightening by treatment with hydrogen peroxide may be necessary before tinting to give an effective colour change.

If the hair has previously been permed or relaxed, care is required as the hair will be fragile showing loss of elasticity, low tensile strength and high porosity.

- At least two deep conditioning treatments are required between perming or relaxing and the application of a permanent colour.
- If the hair is coated with oils or moisturizing products a gentle shampoo may be required before tinting.

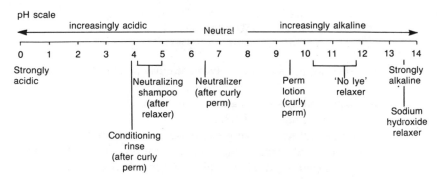

Fig. 16.7 pH values of products used in curly perming and relaxing

- Strand tests taken from several areas of the head are essential before tinting.
- The use of permanent colour as partial colouring, e.g. highlighting, is safer than tinting a whole head especially if pre-lightening is required.

Semi-permanent dyes (nitro dyes)

Strongly coloured semi-permanent dyes may be successfully used on very porous hair because there will be good uptake of the dye. The small dye molecules of semi-permanent dyes will, however, wash out more easily from porous hair.

Temporary dyes (azo dyes)

Temporary colour in the form of mousses, sprays and paints can be successfully applied, particularly in vivid colours.

Vegetable dyes

Henna is often used, though mainly as a conditioner, because the black pigment of Afro hair is too intense for henna to have a marked effect except in bright sunlight, when red highlights are produced.

BLEACHING

The types of bleach available for Afro hair are the same as for European hair (see Chapter 15). In Afro hairdressing, bleaching is mainly used for fashion techniques such as highlighting and tipping. Full head bleaches are rarely carried out and are not advised on hair previously damaged by chemical treatments.

SELF TESTING

1. What precautions are required before carrying out a curly perm? Describe the chemical reactions which take place during the two stages of perming and during neutralizing.
2. Why is conditioning important after a curly perm? What types of conditioners are most suitable?

3. What damage to the hair may occur by (a) over-processing a curly perm (b) overlapping during a retouch perm (c) over-neutralizing?
4. What is meant by a 'no lye' relaxer?
5. What type of chemical reaction takes place during relaxing? What type of linkage replaces cystine linkages in relaxed hair?
6. Why cannot a curly perm be carried out on previously relaxed hair?
7. Why should a neutralizing shampoo be applied with minimal massage after use of a relaxer?
8. Why can a neutralizing shampoo never be used to 'neutralize' a curly perm?
9. What precautions are required before tinting relaxed hair?
10. Why are permanent colours and bleaches often used only to highlight Afro hair?

Notes on Chemicals

Acetic acid	Used as conditioning rinse (vinegar rinse)
Almond oil	Vegetable oil used for hot oil conditioning treatments. Ingredient of control creams
Aluminium chlorhydrate	Astringent in antiperspirant lotions
Amino acids	Units from which proteins are built. Contained in protein hydrolysates
Ammonium carbonate	Alkaline white solid used in paste bleaches to speed the release of oxygen from hydrogen peroxide
Ammonium hydroxide	Alkali used as wetting agent and swelling agent in bleaches, tints and perm lotions to aid penetration of other chemicals into the hairshaft. Catalyst used to speed release of oxygen from hydrogen peroxide during bleaching
Ammonium laurylsulphate	Thick amber coloured liquid anionic detergent. Main ingredient of many shampoos
Ammonium persulphate	Oxidizing agent added to bleaches as a booster
Ammonium thioglycollate	Reducing agent. Active ingredient in perm lotions
Anthraquinones	Semi-permanent dyes (blue)
Apigenin	Active agent in camomile vegetable dyes
Ascorbic acid	Anti-oxidant (reducing agent) used to stop the action of hydrogen peroxide and improve hair condition after bleaching and tinting
Borax (sodium borate)	Used as a mild alkaline rinse for seborrhoea. Added to lacquer-removing

	shampoos. Ingredient of dry powder shampoos
Butane	Propellant for aerosols. Flammable
Calamine (zinc carbonate)	Applied as lotion to ease skin irritation due to positive reaction to dye sensitivity test
Calcium bicarbonate	Cause of temporary hardness in water
Calcium carbonate (limestone)	Deposited as fur or scale in steamers and in shampoo spray heads, etc., when temporary hard water is heated
Calcium hydroxide	Ingredient of 'no-lye' relaxers for Afro hair
Calcium stearate	Lime soap (scum) formed when soap is used in hard water
Calcium sulphate	Cause of permanent hardness in water
Calgon (sodium hexametaphosphate)	Water softener sometimes added to shampoos or used as a rinse after soap shampoo
Camomile	Vegetable dye gives yellow cast to hair
Carbaryl	Insecticide used in lotions to destroy head lice (Prescription required from 1996)
Carbon tetrachloride	Formerly used as wig cleaner
Carbopol	Gelling agent for gel bleaches
Carnauba wax	Ingredient of brilliantines. Vegetable wax from surface of palm leaves
Castor oil	Vegetable oil used in control creams and in manufacture of detergents
Cetrimide (cetyl trimethylammonium bromide)	Quaternary ammonium compound. Cationic detergent and antiseptic. Substantive to hair. Used as medicated shampoo. Main ingredient of cream rinses. Added to many hairdressing products as conditioner
Cetyl alcohol	Emulsifying agent in perm lotions, conditioning creams and cream oxidation dyes
Chlorhexidene	Antiseptic used with alcohol as disinfectant wipe for scissors, curling tongs, etc.
Citric acid	Added to acid-balanced shampoos. Used in rinses to neutralize alkali left on hair after perming, bleaching and tinting
Coconut imidazoline	Detergent in very mild shampoos
Coconut oil	Vegetable oil used in manufacture of soap and soapless detergents
Collodion	Film former to cover dye area in sensitivity test
Copper sulphate	Ingredient of some metallic dyes

Copper sulphide	Metallic sulphide dye
Cysteic acid	Formed in keratin by oxidation of cystine by over-neutralizing a perm or during bleaching
Cysteine	Amino acid formed in hair by reduction of cystine during perming
Cystine	Amino acid in keratin forming a linkage between adjacent polypeptide chains and containing a disulphide bond
Diaminobenzene (para-phenylenediamine)	Permanent oxidation dye (black)
Diaminotoluene (para-toluenediamine)	Permanent oxidation dye (brown)
Dimethyl hydantoin formaldehyde	Plastic resin film former in hair spray and setting lotions
Dimethyl silicone (dimethicone)	Silicone oil (silicone fluid) used in barrier creams, hair sprays and heat setting lotions to produce a water-resistant film. Restructurant to repair split ends. Conditioner in shampoos
Essential oils	Sweet-smelling volatile plant oils used in perfumes
Ethanol (alcohol)	Solvent for resins in hair spray and setting lotions
Formaldehyde	Disinfectant gas produced by heating formalin (formerly used in salon sterilizing cabinets)
Glutaraldehyde	Liquid disinfectant used as bath for tools. Has replaced use of formaldehyde
Glycerol (glycerine)	Emollient used in hand creams. Plasticizer in hair spray. Humectant in conditioners for Afro hair
Glycerol monothioglycollate	Reducing agent in acid perm lotions
Guanidine hydroxide	'No lye' alkaline hair relaxer for Afro hair.
Gum karaya	Gum for setting lotions
Gum tragacanth	Gum for setting lotions
Henna	Permanent vegetable dye (red shades)
Hexachlorophane	Antiseptic in medicated shampoo. Deodorant in antiperspirants
Hydrogen peroxide	Oxidizing agent in bleaches, perm neutralizers and for oxidation of para dyes
Hydrolysed protein	Proteins split into amino acids by

	hydrolysis. (See protein hydrolysates)
Hydroxymethyl imidazoline	Used in acid solution as a hair restructurant
Isopropanol	Solvent for plastic resins in hair sprays and setting lotions
Isopropyl myristate	Plasticizer in hair spray
Jojoba	Liquid (vegetable) wax similar to sebum. Used as conditioner in shampoos
Lactic acid	Weak acid used in acid balanced shampoos
Lanette wax	Synthetic wax (mixture of cetyl and steryl alcohols) used as emulsifying agent
Lanolin	Wax from sheep's wool. Similar to sebum. Added as a conditioner in shampoos and permanent dyes and as a plasticizer in hair sprays
Lanthionine	Amino acid which replaces cystine (disulphide) linkages in keratin after relaxing Afro hair. Lanthionine linkages contain only one sulphur atom
Lauryl diethanolamide	Non-ionic detergent used as foam stabilizer in shampoos
Lawsone	Active ingredient in henna dyes
Lead acetate	A salt used in metallic dyes
Liquid paraffin	Mineral oil used in control creams and in pomades for use in thermal straightening of Afro hair
Magnesium bicarbonate	Cause of temporary hardness in water
Magnesium carbonate (white henna)	White powder used as thickener in powder bleaches
Magnesium sulphate	Cause of permanent hardness in water
Malathion	Insecticide used in lotions to destroy head lice
Methylated spirit	Solvent for resins in hair sprays and setting lotions
Methyl cellulose	Thickener in gel shampoos and gel dressing aids
Methylene Blue	Cationic temporary dye
Methyl thiazolinone	Detergent producing a thick foam in aerosol mousses
Methyl Violet	Cationic temporary dye
Monoethanolamine thioglycollate	Reducing agent used in some perm lotions in place of ammonium thioglycollate
Nipagin	Preservative added to shampoos during

	manufacture to prevent deterioration by bacterial or mould growth
Nitro-phenylenediamine	Semi-permanent dye (yellow)
Olive oil	Vegetable oil used in hot oil treatments
Para-aminobenzoic acid	Active ingredient in sunscreen sprays
Paraffin oil	Mineral oil used in control creams and pomades for thermal straightening of Afro hair
Paraffin wax	Mineral wax used in control creams. Also in pressing creams for Afro hair
Para-hydroxyazobenzene	Azo dye producing temporary colour
Para-phenylenediamine	Permanent oxidation dye (black)
Para-toluenediamine	Permanent oxidation dye (brown)
Petroleum jelly (Vaseline)	Used for basing the scalp during relaxing of Afro hair. Ingredient of solid brilliantine and pomades
Phenolphthalein	Chemical indicator added to neutralizing shampoos to show presence of alkali on the hair by colouring the lather pink
Phosphoric acid	Stabilizer for hydrogen peroxide added during manufacture
Polypeptide chain	Series of amino acids linked by peptide bonds
Polyvinyl acetate (PVA)	Plastic resin film former for hair sprays and setting lotions
Polyvinyl pyrrolidone (PVP)	Plastic resin film former for hair sprays and setting lotions. Humectant and substantive conditioner added to shampoos and perm lotions
Potassium hydroxide	Alkali used in making soft soap shampoos
Potassium oleate	Soft soap used for shampoos
Potassium persulphate	Oxidizing agent added to bleaches as a booster
Propane	Propellant for aerosols. Flammable
Propylene glycol	Humectant used as conditioner in many Afro products. Used as fixative in gel dressing aids
Protein hydrolysates	Substantive conditioners used in pre-perm fillers, perm lotions, shampoos and many other hairdressing preparations (*see* hydrolysed protein)
Quaternary ammonium compounds	Antiseptics and conditioners (*see* cetrimide)

Salicylic acid	Stabilizer for hydrogen peroxide added during manufacture
Selenium sulphide	Active ingredient in anti-dandruff shampoos
Shellac	Natural resin used as film former in lacquer
Silicone oils	See dimethyl silicone
Silver nitrate	A salt used in metallic dyes
Sodium alginate	Thickener for shampoos
Sodium bromate	Oxidizing agent in perm neutralizers
Sodium carbonate	Washing soda. Bath salts
Sodium chloride (common salt)	Regenerates sodium ion exchange resin in water softeners. Used as thickener for soapless shampoos
Sodium formaldehyde sulphoxylate	Reducing agent. Colour remover (stripper) for permanent dyes
Sodium hexametaphosphate	*See* Calgon
Sodium hydroxide (caustic soda)	Caustic alkali (lye) used in relaxers for Afro hair. Used also in manufacture of detergents
Sodium hypochlorite	Bleaching fluid used to clear blood spills
Sodium lauryl ether sulphate	Detergent in clear liquid soapless shampoos
Sodium lauryl sarcosinate	Soapless detergent used in aerosol shampoos
Sodium lauryl sulphate	Detergent used in cream soapless shampoos
Sodium stearate	A hard soap
Sodium sulphide	Used in two application metallic dyes. Also a depilatory
Sodium thiosulphate	Ingredient of hair colour restorers
Sulphonated castor oil (Turkey red oil)	Acts as both a detergent and an oil in conditioning shampoos for dry hair
Sulphonated olive oil	Acts as both a detergent and an oil in conditioning shampoos for dry hair
Sulphuric acid	Used in making soapless detergents
Tartaric acid	Added to temporary acid dyes to make the dye cling to the hair
Terbinafine	Drug used to treat cases of ringworm
Tetrachloroethane	Grease solvent used for cleaning wigs
Thioglycollic acid	Used in the manufacture of perm lotion
Trichlorocarbanilide	Antiseptic used in medicated shampoos
Triethanolamine	An alkali used in the manufacture of soap and soapless detergents

Triethanolamine lauryl sulphate	Detergent used in clear liquid soapless shampoos
Turkey red oil	*See* sulphonated castor oil
Urea	Used in acid perm lotions to aid penetration of the lotion into the hair shaft
Vaseline	*See* petroleum jelly
Zeolite	A natural resin formerly used in water softeners
Zinc carbonate	*See* calamine
Zinc pyrithione (zinc omadine)	Active ingredient in anti-dandruff shampoos

GLOSSARY

Accelerator	Infra-red lamps used as source of heat for drying hair or to speed chemical processing
Acid	A compound producing hydrogen ions and having a pH of less than 7
Acid mantle	Natural acidity of the skin due to sweat and sebum giving the skin a pH of 5−6
Afro hair	Typical tightly curled hair of people of Afro origin
Albino	Person with no pigment in hair, skin or eyes due to rare genetic defect
Alkali	Compound producing hydroxyl ions and having a pH of between 7 and 14
Allergen	Substance causing an allergic reaction
Allergy	Sensitivity of the skin to certain chemicals which cause dermatitis
Alopecia	General term for baldness
Alpha-helix	Coiled spring arrangement of polypeptide chains in keratin
Alpha-keratin	Keratin in an unstretched state
Ampere	Unit of intensity or size of an electric current
Ampholyte	Detergent which is cationic in acid solution and anionic in alkaline solution
Anagen	Period of active growth of hair in a follicle lasting from two to seven years
Anionic detergent	Detergent producing ions carrying a negative electrical charge
Antibiotic	Drug used to fight bacterial infection
Antibody	Substance produced in the blood to fight virus infections
Antioxidant	Reducing agent used to halt oxidation after using an oxidation dye, a bleach or neutralizing a perm

Antiseptic	Substance used on skin to inhibit growth of bacteria
Apocrine gland	Sweat gland found in armpit area. Bacterial decomposition of the sweat leads to body odour
Arrector pili muscle	Muscle attached to a hair follicle. Contraction of this muscle makes hair stand erect
Astringent	Substance which has a tightening effect on the skin
Atom	Smallest part of an element. Atoms join chemically to form molecules
Azo dye	Type of temporary dye
Basing (scalp)	Application of protective oil to the scalp before relaxing Afro hair
Beta-keratin	Keratin in a stretched state
Booster (bleach)	Persulphates added to bleach to provide extra oxygen
Bound water	Water in cortex which enters hydrogen bonds allowing increased ability of hair to stretch
Capillary rise	Ability of liquids to rise up through narrow spaces
Catagen	Period of change from active growth to resting stage of follicles in growth cycle of a hair, lasting about two weeks
Catalyst	Substance which speeds up a chemical reaction while remaining unchanged itself
Cationic conditioner	Positively charged conditioner which is attracted to negative charges in the hair, e.g. cetrimide
Cationic detergent	Detergent producing ions with a positive electrical charge
Club hair	Hair detached from base of follicle during catagen
Cohesive set	Stretching wet hair, and drying in stretched state, e.g. roller setting and blow drying
Compound	Chemical consisting of two or more elements
Condensation	Water deposited when warm moist air meets a cold surface
Cortex	Fibrous layer of hair between cuticle and medulla containing granules of pigment melanin
Cow lick	Unusual pattern of strong hair growth in which a small section of hair grows in a different direction to the rest of the hair on the front hair line
Cross linkages	Chemical bridges in keratin connecting adjacent polypeptide chains
Cuticle	Outer layer of hair consisting of overlapping scales

Dandruff	Over-production and shedding of skin scales from the scalp
Depilatory	Chemical hair remover
Dermal papilla	Projections of the dermis into the epidermis along the junction between the two and also at the base of the hair follicles (*see* hair papilla)
Dermis	Lower of the two layers of the skin
Detergent	A substance used with water to clean surfaces
Disinfectant	Chemical used to destroy bacteria
Disulphide bond	Chemical bond in cystine linkage of keratin and containing two sulphur atoms
Double crown	Unusual pattern of hair growth in which hairs radiate from two points at the top of the head. Normally only one crown is present
Earth wire	Electrical safety device to protect people from shock by carrying a dangerous current from a faulty appliance to earth. Normally carries no current
Eccrine glands	Sweat glands found in most parts of the skin
Effleurage	A stroking movement of massage
Elasticity	Ability of a hair to be stretched and return to its original length when the stretching force is removed
Elastic limit	Point in stretching when a hair will no longer return to its original length when released
Element	A substance which cannot be split into any simpler substances and contains only one type of atom
Emollient	Substance applied to hair to prevent moisture loss from the hair, so keeping the hair soft and pliable
Emulsifying agent (emulsifier)	Substance used to emulsify oil and water; for example, shampoo is an emulsifying agent used to remove grease from hair by making an oil-in-water emulsion
Emulsion	Droplets of one liquid suspended in another liquid, e.g. oil in water or water in oil.
Epicranial aponeurosis	A sheet of tendon covering the top of the head and with the skin above it forming the scalp
Epidermis	The upper of the two layers of the skin
Erythema	Redness caused by increased blood flow to the skin
Essential oils	Sweet-smelling volatile plant oils used in perfumes
Filler	Lotion designed to equalize porosity in the hair

	shaft before chemical processing, e.g. pre-perm filler
Follicle	A tubular downgrowth into the dermis of epidermal cells from which a hair grows
Folliculitis	Bacterial infection of a hair follicle
Fragilitas crinium	Split ends caused by physical or chemical damage to the hair shaft
Frictions	Massage involving small circular kneading movements used during shampooing and applying scalp lotions
Fungi	Plants with no green colouring matter such as those causing ringworm
Fuse	Protective device in an electrical circuit designed to melt if the current becomes too large thus breaking the circuit and protecting wiring from overheating
Germinal matrix	Part of the follicle where hair growth takes place (also called hair root)
Germinating layer	Lower layer of the epidermis consisting of actively dividing cells
Gland	An organ in the body producing a substance which is secreted or expelled from the gland, e.g. sweat glands secrete sweat and sebaceous glands secrete sebum
Glare	A bright light shining into the eyes and causing discomfort
Hair line	Junction between the scalp hair and the skin of the face and neck
Hair papilla	Part of the dermis holding blood capillaries at the base of a hair follicle and surrounded by epidermal cells of the hair bulb from which the hair grows
Hair root	Bulb-shaped group of cells from which the hair grows at the base of the follicle
Hair shaft	The part of a hair above the surface of the skin
Hair spray	Aerosol product containing plastic resins dissolved in alcohol. Sprayed on dry hair to hold the hair in position after styling (see also lacquer)
Halitosis	Unpleasant breath
Hard water	Water containing dissolved salts, usually calcium or magnesium salts, which produces a scum with soap before forming a lather
High frequency current	Rapidly alternating current used to increase blood circulation to the scalp

Horny layer	Upper layer of the epidermis consisting of protective layer of dead cells
Humectant	Substance applied to hair to attract moisture to the cortex
Humidity	Amount of moisture present in the air
Hydrogen bonds	Weak chemical bonds in keratin which limit the stretching of a hair
Hydrolysis	Chemical reaction where a substance is broken down by the addition of the elements of water, e.g. relaxing Afro hair by use of sodium hydroxide
Hydrophilic	Refers to a molecule or ion which is water-loving
Hydrophobic	Refers to a molecule or ion which is water-hating
Hygrometer	Instrument used to measure relative humidity
Hygroscopic	Absorbs moisture from the air
Hyperaemia	Increased blood flow to the skin producing redness of the skin (erythema)
Impetigo	Bacterial skin infection with small blisters followed by yellow crusts
Infection	Attack on body by disease-causing micro-organisms
Infectious	Describes a disease which can be passed from person to person
Infestation	Attack on body by small animal parasites, e.g. lice
Infra-red rays	Invisible rays producing heat
Inner root sheath	Protective sheath round the hair inside the follicle
Ion	Part of an atom with a positive or negative charge
Keloid	Scar tissue raised above the surface of the skin
Keratin	The protein of hair, nails and the outer layer of the epidermis
Keratinization	The hardening of keratin during its development
Keratolytic	A substance which breaks down keratin
Lacquer (Hair Spray)	Aerosol product, originally containing shellac but now containing plastic resins dissolved to alcohol. Designed to be sprayed on to dry hair to hold the hair in position after styling
Lanugo hair	Very fine hair on the skin of a foetus
Latent heat	Heat required to change a liquid to a vapour, e.g. evaporation of sweat takes latent heat from the skin (also heat given out when a vapour changes to a liquid)
Lice	Insects living on the head or body and taking nourishment by drawing blood from the skin

Lime scale	Deposit of calcium carbonate in kettles, etc., when temporary hard water is heated
Lime soap	Scum of calcium soap formed when soap is used in hard water
Malpighian layer	Lower living layers of the epidermis
Medulla	The central core of a hair
Melanin	Black or brown pigment in hair and skin
Melanocytes	Pigment-producing cells in the germinating layer of the epidermis
Micro-organisms	Living organisms which are too small to be seen by the naked eye, e.g. bacteria, viruses and some fungi
Mineral oils	Oils originating in the ground, e.g. paraffin oil and petroleum jelly
Molecule	Smallest part of a compound, consisting of two or more atoms
Monilethrix	Defect of hair leading to beaded hair shaft
Mousse	A foaming aerosol product used as a setting or styling aid
Mycelium	A mass of thread-like fungus cells
Nascent oxygen	Newly formed oxygen (e.g. from the breakdown of hydrogen peroxide) which is a more powerful bleaching agent than atmospheric oxygen
Neutralization	The chemical reaction between an acid and alkali to form a salt and water
Neutralizing	A hairdressing term for the oxidation process to rebuild cystine linkages after perming (not true chemical neutralization)
Neutralizing shampoo	An acid shampoo designed to chemically neutralize alkali left on the hair after relaxing Afro hair
Nit	Egg of a louse
Nitro dye	A semi-permanent dye
Organic compound	A substance containing carbon atoms and obtained from a living source
Outer root sheath	The outer walls of a hair follicle
Overloading	Attempting, by use of too many appliances in a circuit, to pass a greater current through the circuit than that for which it was designed so causing the fuse to 'blow'
Oxidation	A chemical reaction involving the addition of oxygen to a substance

Oxidizing agent	A chemical, e.g. hydrogen peroxide, which gives oxygen to another substance during a chemical reaction
Para dye	Synthetic permanent oxidation dye
Parasite	A living organism which lives on or in another organism from which it takes nourishment
Pathogen	A micro-organism which causes disease
Pediculosis	Infestation by lice
Pediculus capitis	Head louse
Peptide bond	Chemical bond between amino acids in a polypeptide chain
Peroxometer	An instrument (type of hydrometer) used to measure the strength of hydrogen peroxide
Petrissage	Main movement of scalp massage (kneading action)
pH	Symbol for hydrogen ion concentration indicating degree of acidity or alkalinity of a substance
Pheomelanin	Red and yellow pigments of hair
Pityriasis capitis	Dandruff
Plasticizer	Chemical used as softener of plastic resins e.g. isopropyl myristate softens the film of lacquers
Porosity (hair)	Ability of hair to absorb liquids
Postiche	False hair pieces attached to the natural hair to create more elaborate styles
Pre-perm lotion	Lotion used before perming to even out porosity of the hairshaft
Propellant	Volatile substance, e.g. butane, which creates a vapour pressure to force the product from an aerosol container
Protein	Substance consisting of chemically linked amino acids, e.g. hair keratin
Protofibril	Finest fibre of the cortex consisting of three coiled polypeptide chains
Psoriasis	Non-infectious skin condition with characteristic thick silvery scales sometimes on the scalp
Pustule	A raised spot on the skin containing pus
Quasi-permanent dye	Mixture of semi-permanent and permanent dyes requiring a skin test before application
Radiation	Wave-motion by which heat travels from a hot object in straight lines through space
Reducing agent	A chemical which adds hydrogen (or takes oxygen away) during a chemical reaction, e.g. ammonium thioglycollate in perm lotion
Reduction	A chemical reaction in which hydrogen is added

	to a substance (or oxygen is taken away)
Relaxer	A chemical used to straighten tightly curled hair, e.g. sodium hydroxide
Restructurant	Lotion used on hair to repair damage particularly to internal structure
Ring main circuit	Electrical circuit in the form of a ring into which power sockets can be fitted
Ringworm	Infectious fungal disease of the hair and skin
Sabouraud-Rousseau test	Name given to the skin test used to detect allergic reaction to para dyes (see also skin test)
Salt	Substance formed by the neutralization of an acid by an alkali
Salt linkage	Electrostatic bond between an acid group and an amino group in adjacent polypeptide chains in hair keratin
Saponification	Process by which soap is manufactured
Scalp	Consists of the epicranial aponeurosis and its covering skin with the scalp hair
Sebaceous cyst	A sac forming a small raised lump on the scalp due to blockage of the opening of a sebaceous gland
Sebaceous gland	Gland attached to a hair follicle secreting an oily substance called sebum
Seborrhoea	Overactivity of the sebaceous glands resulting in greasy hair and skin
Sebum	The oily secretion of the sebaceous gland
Short circuit	Surge of current usually caused by worn insulation, enabling a live wire to touch either a neutral or earth wire and resulting in a blown fuse
Skin test	Test carried out 24–48 hours before intention to apply a para dye, to ensure that the client is not allergic to the dye
Slithering	A sliding movement which may cause damage to the hair cuticle during razor cutting
Soapless shampoo	A shampoo that contains a synthetic detergent rather than soap
Solute/solvent/ solution	A solute is a substance which dissolves in a liquid, called the solvent, so forming a solution
Stabilizer	An acid added to hydrogen peroxide to prevent premature release of oxygen during storage
Static electricity	The build-up of an electrical charge by friction, e.g. on dry hair by brushing
Sterilization	Complete destruction of all living organisms on an object

Stripper	Colour remover for permanent dyes
Subcutaneous	Underneath the skin
Substantive conditioner	Conditioner with a positive electrical charge which is attracted to negative acid groups in the hair shaft
Surface tension	Forces in water causing contraction of the surface so that water forms spherical droplets which do not spread easily over other surfaces to wet them
Surfactants	Detergents which act as wetting agents by lowering surface tension of water (also called surface active agents)
Tapotement	A tapping or patting movement of massage rarely used on the scalp
Telogen	The resting stage in the growth cycle of a hair follicle lasting three to four months
Tendon	Non-elastic tissue attaching a muscle to a bone
Tensile strength	The force required to break a hair by stretching or the weight that a hair will support before breaking
Terminal hair	The coarse hair found on the scalp, and after puberty in beard area and chest of men and in underarm and pubic areas
Texture (hair)	The feel of hair depending on diameter, the amount of moisture in the cortex and roughness of the cuticle
Tinea capitis	Ringworm of the scalp
Toner	Colourant used after bleaching
Traction alopecia	Baldness caused by repeated tension on the hair
Trichorrhexis nodosa	Non-infectious hair condition recognized by nodes or small split swellings on the hair shaft and caused by physical or chemical damage
Ultra-violet rays	Rays produced by a mercury vapour lamp and used in a salon ultra-violet cabinet to keep tools germ free
Vellus hair	Fine downy hair found on most parts of the skin
Verruca	A wart
Vibrations (massage)	Scalp massage by use of a trembling movement of the fingers
Vibro massage	Use of an electrical appliance to massage the scalp
Virgin hair	Hair untreated by chemicals
Viruses	Micro-organisms causing diseases such as AIDS, colds, cold sores and influenza

Volt	A unit of electrical pressure
Wattage	A measurement of the power of an appliance, or the rate at which the appliance uses electricity
Wetting agent	A substance, e.g. a detergent, which lowers the surface tension of water
Whorl	Unusual circular pattern of hair growth at the nape.
Widow's peak	Pattern of hair growth in which the hair line forms a point at the centre of the forehead

INDEX